IMMUNOLOGY AND IMMUNE SYSTEM DISORDERS

LUPUS RENAL INVOLVEMENT

A CASE-BASED ATLAS

IMMUNOLOGY AND IMMUNE SYSTEM DISORDERS

Additional books in this series can be found on Nova's website under the Series tab.

Additional e-books in this series can be found on Nova's website under the e-book tab.

IMMUNOLOGY AND IMMUNE SYSTEM DISORDERS

LUPUS RENAL INVOLVEMENT

A CASE-BASED ATLAS

GYL EANES BARROS SILVA, MD, PHD
ROBERTO SILVA COSTA, MD, PHD
MÁRCIO DANTAS, MD, PHD
NATALINO SALGADO FILHO, MD, PHD
AND
STANLEY DE ALMEIDA ARAUJO, MD

NOVA BIOMEDICAL
New York

Library of Congress Cataloging-in-Publication Data

ISBN: 978-1-63463-834-0
Library of Congress Control Number: 2015949948

Published by Nova Science Publishers, Inc. † New York

Contents

Preface		**vii**
Glossary of Pathologic Descriptive Terms and Patterns		**ix**
Chapter 1	Introduction	**1**
Chapter 2	Class I and II	**7**
Chapter 3	Class III and IV	**13**
Chapter 4	Class V	**23**
Chapter 5	Class VI	**29**
Chapter 6	Tubulointerstitial Lesions	**31**
Chapter 7	Vascular Lesions	**35**
Chapter 8	Lupus Overlap Diseases	**43**
Chapter 9	Other Glomerular Lesions	**49**
Chapter 10	Lupus and Drugs	**53**
References		**57**
Authors' Contact Information		**61**
Index		**63**

Preface

Renal disease, in particular glomerulonephritis, afflicts three fourths of patients with SLE. Although the currently used classification of lupus nephritis is based exclusively on classical glomerular nephritis, it has been described as lupus-unrelated renal injury (drug toxicity, infection, others glomerulonephritis), lupus-associated mechanisms that are not part of the current classification (podocytopathies, thrombotic microangiopathy, vasculopathy, vasculitis, non-inflammatory necrotizing vasculopathy, rhabdomyolysis and others), amyloidosis, renal injury due to concomitant disease (for example, hypertension and diabetes mellitus), etc. Therefore, the correct diagnosis of renal lupus involvement can only be diagnosed by renal biopsy.

This book is a histopathology case-based atlas with contributions from several authors, it intends to fill a gap in literature.

The cases obtained have been collected from patient material from several institutions, including (1) The Renal Pathology Laboratory, Department of Pathology, Ribeirão Preto Medical School, University of São Paulo, Brazil (2) The Renal Pathology Laboratory, Pathology Service, University Hospital of Federal University of Maranhão, Brazil (3) Department of Pathology, Federal University of Minas Gerais, Brazil.

Recommendations for reporting a renal biopsy in a patient with lupus nephritis, the standard definitions that should be applied to renal biopsy interpretation, correlation of the pathologic findings with clinical history and prognosis were also provided. Each case consists of typical histology images, a brief history, diagnosis, discussion, and pearls and pitfalls.

We hope that this revision, which evolved under the auspices of the Brazilian Renal Club, will contribute to further advancement of the spectrum of renal diseases associated with Lupus.

The audiences for the publication are pathologists, nephrologists, rheumatologists, or are interested in learning more about Lupus and Lupus Nephritis.

Glossary of Pathologic Descriptive Terms and Patterns

Crescent (extracapillary proliferation) - Proliferation of cells (>2 cell layers) in the Bowman's space, occupying 25% or more of glomerular capsular circumference.

Cellular crescent – Crescent with cells and no fibrosis.

Diffuse – Involving 50% or more of glomeruli.

Double contours – Duplication of glomerular basement membrane separated by clear zone on silver or PAS stains.

Endocapillary proliferation (hypercellularity) – Increased numbers of intracapillary cells (mesangial cells, endothelial cells and infiltrating leukocytes) causing narrowing of the glomerular capillary lumina.

Fibrinoid necrosis – disruption of GBM, cells and matrix associated with deposition of fibrin.

Fibrocellular crescent - Mixture of cellular and fibrous component.

Fibrous crescent – Predominantly fibrous tissue in urinary space

Fibrous adhesion/synechia: abnormal attachment of glomerular tuft to Bowman capsule.

Focal – Involving less than 50% of glomeruli.

Global – involving the entire glomerular tuft (> 50% in lupus).

Hyaline thrombus – Eosinophilic, homogeneous, rounded aggregates in glomerular capillaries due to immune complex deposition.

Intramembranous – Within the glomerular basement membrane.

Karyorrhexias – Apoptotic, pyknotic, and fragmented nuclei.

Membranoproliferative – Combined capillary wall thickening with prominent double contour and mesangial or endocapillary hypercellularity.

Mesangial hypercellularity – At least three mesangial cells per mesangial area away from the vascular pole in a section of 2-3μm.

Sclerosis – Obliteration of capillary lumen by increased of matrix (glomerular scarring).

Segmental – Involving less than half of the glomerular tuft.

Subendothelial – Space between the endothelium and the glomerular basement membrane.

Supepithelial – Space between pocytes and the glomerular basement membrane.

Wire-loops – thickened glomerular capillary wall with rigid appearance due to large subendothelial immune deposits

Chapter 1

Introduction

Concept of Lupus

Systemic Lupus Erythematosus (SLE) is a systemic autoimmune disease of unknown etiology, affecting multiple organs, including the kidney.

Lupus Nephritis

- Two types of renal involvement have been described: lupus nephritis (LN) (mediated by immune complexes) and non-LN (not mediated by immune complexes). See Table 1.
- Compartments affected: glomerulus (included in World Health Organization [WHO] and International Society of Nephrology/Renal Pathology Society [ISN/RPS] classification), tubules, interstitium, arteries, veins, and peritubular capillaries (not included in the current classifications).
- Silent LN: glomerular deposition of immune complexes and microscopic abnormalities, but no clinical changes.
- Highly variable clinical status: ranging from asymptomatic hematuria and/or proteinuria to nephrotic syndrome, and development of rapidly progressive glomerulonephritis.
- LN is an important cause of morbidity and mortality in lupus patients. Along with sepsis, it is the leading cause of death in SLE.

- Survival at 10 years for lupus patients without nephritis is 80%, and 65% for those with nephritis.
- LN is more prevalent and severe in children, men, and individuals of African descent.
- LN can occur concomitantly, precede (by months or years), or follow (by months or years) the diagnosis of the disease. Diagnostic confirmation of suspected cases of lupus is common after biopsy demonstrates morphological findings and immunopathological characteristics. Quite often, classes II and V precede serological changes and extra-renal manifestations of SLE by months or years. At diagnosis, 50% of patients with lupus have renal lesions.
- The following renal criteria can be considered: persistent proteinuria ≥ 500 mg/day or 3+ by dipstick, or cell casts of any type, if other causes are ruled out. Therefore, renal biopsy is not necessary to establish the diagnosis, but is performed to define the quality and severity of renal injury, and is a guide for treatment. For diagnostic criteria, see Table 2.
- Currently, according to the Systemic Lupus International Collaborating Clinics (SLICC) group, the diagnosis of SLE can be made only with a biopsy compatible with LN and positive serology (antinuclear antibodies or anti-double-stranded DNA antibodies.
- Renal involvement will occur in 2/3 of patients at some point (>90% in studies with electron microscopy and with serial biopsies). Renal survival at 10 years is 75%.

Renal Biopsy in Lupus

Indications for Renal Biopsy in Lupus:

1) Lupus patient without histological diagnosis of LN.
    - Appearance of any marker of renal disease: hematuria, proteinuria, nephrotic syndrome, or increased creatinine levels.
2) Lupus patient with histological diagnosis of LN.
    - Evaluate the effectiveness of treatment and the need for continuation or modification.
    - Suspicion for class transformation.
3) Patient without diagnosis of Lupus.

- -Confirm the diagnosis in a patient with renal changes and antinuclear or anti-double stranded (anti-dsDNA) antibodies.

Purpose of Biopsy:

- Establish the extent and severity of renal injury.
- -Determine the class (I-IV).
- Determine the activity of glomerulonephritis.
- -Evaluate the therapeutic response.
- Confirm the diagnosis of lupus.

Important Information provided by Biopsy:

1) Prognostic information (a biopsy is the best prognostic predictor of LN).

- Class:
- II and V are better than III and IV.
- Class information from the first biopsy is more important. Value reduced in subsequent biopsies.
- Quantity of subendothelial deposits.
- Related to the degree of endocapillary proliferation and the presence of necrosis.
- Activity and Chronicity Index.
- Reproducibility questionable, large interobserver variability.
- Prognostic value greater with comparison of biopsies from the same patient.
- Worst prognosis: indices of activity >12 and chronicity >3.

2) Important information for clinical management: class, activity and chronicity indices, and interstitial and vascular damage.

Frequency of Classes in Biopsies:

Class I: 1%
Class II: 10-15%
Class III: 15-25%
Class IV: 40-60%
Class V: 10-15%

Table 1. Forms of Renal involvement in Lupus

• **Mediated by immune complexes**

Glomerular
• Lupus nephritis (Classes I to VI - WHO or ISN/RPS)
• Tubulointerstitial nephritis**
• Vascular lesions
• Deposition of non-complicated immune complexes
• Lupus vasculopathy
• Necrotizing arteritis
• Thrombotic microangiopathy
    • With APS
    • Without APS

• **Not mediated by immune complexes**

Podocytopathies
  • Minimal lesion disease
  • Focal and segmental glomerulosclerosis
  • Collapsing glomerulosclerosis
Hypertensive nephrosclerosis
  Amyloidosis
  Acute allergic interstitial nephritis
  Acute tubular necrosis due to rhabdomyolysis

• **Nephritis caused by other diseases associated with lupus**
HIV ANCA-related vasculitis Overlap Syndrome: Scleroderma and SLE*** IgA nephropathy DM - induced by immunosuppressants Other glomerulopathies: Primary IgA Nephropathy, Sarcoidosis
• **Drug-induced secondary lupus nephritis**

* For complete list, see Table 2. ** Usually associated with glomerular injury. *** Commonly associated with Thrombotic Microangiopathy.

Table 2. Criteria of the American Rheumatism Association for the diagnosis of LUPUS

- Malar rash
- Discoid rash
- Photosensitivity
- Oral ulcers
- Non-deforming arthritis
- Serositis
- Kidney disease
- Involvement of the central nervous system
- Hematological changes
- Immunological changes
- Positive antinuclear antibody

Types of class Transformations:

– Spontaneously or after treatment (more common).

II↔III, IV

III↔IV

V↔IV

– Signs of transformation for proliferative classes.

A significant increase of proteinuria or worsening of renal function.

– Signs of transformation for non-proliferative classes.

An improvement in proteinuria or renal function.

Chapter 2

Class I and II

Class I (or Ib WHO)

Clinical:

- Benign course with mild-to-moderate renal changes, such as microscopic hematuria or mild proteinuria. Renal function is preserved.
- Some patients can have concomitant active systemic lupus.

Morphology:

- Light microscopy (LM) is normal. Immunofluorescence (IF) and electron microscopy (EM) show mesangial deposits.
- Note that class Ia of the WHO classification (modified, 1995), which corresponds to the original WHO class I (1974 and 1982), was deleted in the classification by ISN/RPS. To understand the differences among the lupus classification systems adopted over time, see Table 3.

Table 3. A comparison table among different classification systems adopted over time

Classes	WHO (Original)	WHO (1994)	ISN/RPS
I	**Normal glomeruli**	**Normal glomerulus (LM, IF, EM)**	**Minimum Mesangial Changes**
			Normal glomeruli by optical microscopy; however, with deposits by IF and/or EM
II	**Pure Mesangial Disease**	**Pure mesangial changes**	**Proliferative mesangial changes**
	a) OM normal, deposits by IF and/or EM b) Mesangial	c) LM normal, mesangial deposits by IF or EM d) Mesangial Hypercellularity and deposits by IF or EM	Mesangial Hypercellularity of any degree, or expansion of mesangial matrix by LM, with immune or mesangial deposits. There may be few and isolated epithelial and subendothelial deposits visible by IF or EM, but with normal LM.
III	**Focal Proliferative GN**	**Segmental and focal glomerulonephritis**	**Focal Lupus Glomerulonephritis**
	< 50% of the glomeruli	a) Active necrotizing lesions b) Active sclerosing lesions c) Sclerosing lesions	Focal, segmental, or global GN, endo- or extracapillary, active or inactive, which involves <50% of the glomeruli with focal subendothelial deposits, with or without mesangial changes **Class III (A)** - with active lesions: focal proliferative GN; **Class III (A/C)** - with active and chronic lesions: focal proliferative and sclerosing GN; **Class III (C)** - chronic and inactive lesions with glomerular sclerosis: focal sclerosing GN.
IV	**Diffuse Proliferative GN**	**Diffuse Glomerulonephritis (serious mesangial, endocapillary, or mesangiocapillary proliferation, and/or extensive subendothelial deposits)**	**Diffuse Lupus Glomerulonephritis**

Classes	WHO (Original)	WHO (1994)	ISN/RPS
	≥ 50% of glomeruli	a) Without additional lesions b) With active necrotizing lesions c) With active sclerosing lesions d) With sclerosing lesions	Diffuse GN, segmental or global, endo- or extracapillary, active or inactive, involving >50% of the glomeruli with diffuse subendothelial deposits, with or without mesangial changes. This class is divided into diffuse segmental (IV-S), where more than 50% of glomeruli have segmental lesions, diffuse and global (IV-G), where more than 50% of glomeruli have global lesions. **Class IV-S (A)** - Diffuse proliferative segmental GN, with active lesions. **Class IV-G (A)** - Diffuse global proliferative GN, with active lesions. **Class IV-S (A/C)** - Proliferative and diffuse sclerosing segmental GN, with active chronic lesions. **Class IV-S (C)** - GN with chronic and inactive lesions with segmental sclerosis. **Class IV-G (C)** - GN with chronic and inactive lesions with global sclerosis.
V	**Membranous GN**	**Membranous Glomerulonephritis**	**Lupus Membranous Glomerulonephritis**
		a) Pure Membranous Glomerulonephritis b) Associated with class II (a or b) lesions	Presence of global or segmental subepithelial deposits, or their morphological sequelae by LM, IF, or EM, with or without mesangial changes. May occur in association with classes III and IV.
VI		**Advanced Sclerosing Glomerulonephritis**	**Glomerulonephritis with advanced sclerosis**
			>90% of the glomeruli have global sclerosis, without residual inflammatory activity

Class II

Clinical:

- Mild clinical manifestations, such as mild hematuria and/or proteinuria (generally <1 g/24 h). There is no nephrotic syndrome. Renal failure is very rare.
- Serology strongly positive in only a quarter of the cases.
- Classes I and II correspond to 70% of the biopsies of patients with silent lupus.

Morphology:

- Class II changes are visible on LM. It is characterized by mesangial hypercellularity, defined as three or more cells per mesangial axis in thin (2–3 μm thick) sections in areas away from the vascular pole, or by deposition of matrix. Although not very common, visible mesangial deposits can be found.
- In some cases, sparse subendothelial or subepithelial deposits can be seen, but only on IF and on EM. Presence of subendothelial deposits detectable by LM indicates, very probably, an unsampled focal proliferative lesion, or the possibility of imminent evolution to class III or IV. The presence of glomerular sclerosis (segmental or global) is indicative of a scar of a proliferative lesion, class III or IV, and is incompatible with the diagnosis of class II. Such cases should receive the designation "C," for chronic injuries. Lesions in other compartments are infrequent.

Case: A 27-year-old woman, with diagnosis of SLE followed by rheumatology for seven years, presented with proteinuria of 0.5-1 g/ 24 h in recent months. Laboratory exams reveal absence of urinary sediment and negativity for anti-DNA.

Biopsy: GLOMERULI: 11 glomeruli, the majority only with mild mesangial hypercellularity. TUBULE-INTERSTITIUM: within normal limits. BLOOD VESSELS: within normal limits. IMMUNOFLUORESCENCE: moderate positive mesangial staining for IgA, IgG, C3, and C1q. Diagnosis: mesangial changes compatible with LN class II.

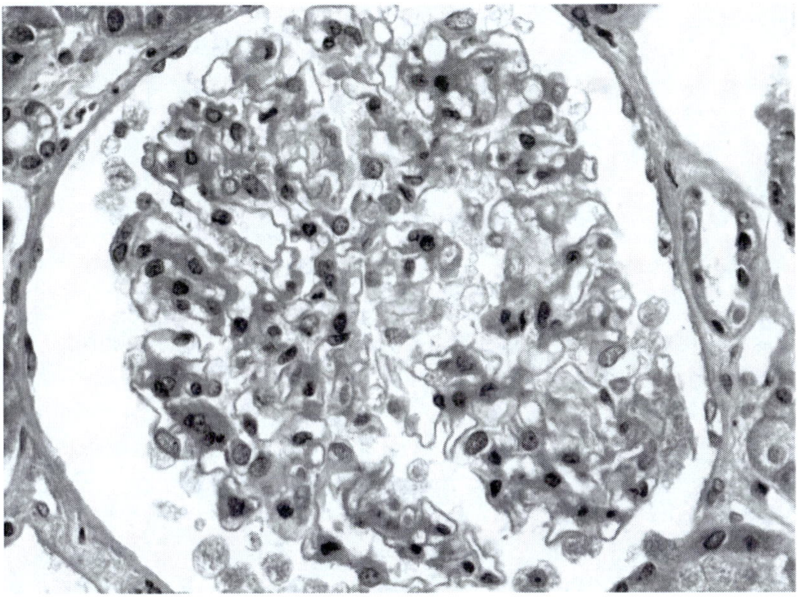

Figure 1. Masson's trichrome: slight increase in mesangial cellularity (>2 cells per mesangial axis), without restriction of capillary light.

Figure 2. IgG: Global and granular, staining in a purely mesangial pattern.

Histological Note:

- The presence of subendothelial deposits, by LM or IF (extension of mesangial staining to the loops), is incompatible with the diagnosis of class II. The possibility of a proliferative class must be seriously considered.

Differential Diagnosis:

The differential diagnosis includes all conditions where immunofluorescence displays a mesangial pattern, mainly primary IgA nephropathy (NIgA). In the last case, the IgA is the dominant, or at least co-dominant, immunoglobulin. In 85% of lupus cases, the predominant immunoglobulin is IgG. Lambda light chain predominates over kappa in 67% of NIgA, versus 29% in lupus. Also, only 10% of NIgA cases present as positive for C1q, generally with lower intensity than in lupus. In addition, in NIgA, the deposition is concentrated in the paramesangial area, while in lupus the distribution is diffuse. Other diseases that must be differentiated are membranoproliferative glomerulonephritis or post-infectious glomerulonephritis in resolving stages of disease. Similar to lupus, these diseases are also hypocomplementemic.

Therapeutic:

- **General measures in treatment of LN:** It is recommended that all patients with LN receive therapy containing hydroxychloroquine. All patients with proteinuria greater than 0.5g/24 h must receive medication for blockade of the renin-angiotensin system, either angiotensin-converting enzyme inhibitors or angiotensin receptor blockers. The use of statins is recommended when low-density lipoprotein cholesterol levels are above 100 mg/dL.
- **Classes I and II:** treatment with immunosuppressive drugs is not required. The treatment consists of general measures, described above, with appropriate monitoring and evaluation for emergence of signs that are suggestive of activity or change of histological class.

Chapter 3

Class III and IV

Proliferative Classes

Class III (Focal LN)

Clinical:

- More aggressive than class II. The clinical history is similar to class IV and, for many, is synonymous with class IV. Half the cases have active urinary sediment, and 25-50% have proteinuria (> 1/3 nephrotic level). Renal failure occurs in 10-25% of the cases. Systemic arterial hypertension affects > 1/3 of the patients. More than half present with hypocomplementemia and/or anti-DNA antibodies.
- Patients with class III have 75% renal survival in 5 years.
- The pathologic features are very similar to those present in class IV, but more than 50% of glomeruli are affected.

Class IV (Diffuse LN)

Clinical:

- Severe clinical course, characterized by nephrotic syndrome and active urinary sediment. Proteinuria is found in virtually all of the cases, with 50% at nephrotic levels. In 3/4 cases, the urine sediment is

active. At the time of biopsy, half of the class IV cases show some degree of renal insufficiency. Anti-DNA antibody-positive and hypocomplementemia: 50-90%.
- If untreated, the patient has a high probability of progression to renal failure (30% of renal survival in 5 years)
- The lesions may be predominantly chronic, sometimes without any sign of activity, leading to progressive renal failure.

Morphology:

- The same lesions are found in both proliferative classes, differing only in the number of glomeruli affected; in the focal class, less than 50% of the glomeruli are affected, whereas in the diffuse one, 50% or more are affected.
- Class III and IV hold subclasses, depending on the presence of active and chronic lesions: A (only active lesions), C (only chronic lesion), and A/C (presence of active and chronic lesions). Class IV is also subdivided into S (segmental lesions) and G (global lesions). In class III, the lesions are almost always segmental.
- The morphological glomerular patterns found in classes III and IV are: endocapillary proliferative lesions (most common), membrane proliferative, extracapillary proliferative (crescentic), and subendothelial deposition without massive proliferation. For this reason the ISN/RPS classification uses the terms “focal LN” and "diffuse LN", instead of "focal proliferative glomerulonephritis" and "diffuse proliferative glomerulonephritis."
- A small amount of subepithelial deposits may be present. The majority of vascular lesions related to lupus, in particular the more serious, are found in class IV.
- Changes present in proliferative classes are divided into active and chronic lesions.

Active lesions:

1. Subendothelial deposits: wire loop (deposits with thickening of the glomerular basement membrane [GBM]) or hyaline thrombi (large intracapillary deposits).
2. Endocapillary proliferation: proliferation of mesangial and endothelial cells with reduction of the lumen of the peripheral capillary loop.

3. Leukocyte infiltration: neutrophils, monocytes, and lymphocytes.
4. Fibrinoid necrosis of glomerular tuft: characterized by deposition of fibrin, rupture of GBM or formation of gaps, neutrophil apoptosis (pyknosis and karyorrhexis).
5. Extracapillary proliferation (crescents): the result from the proliferation of parietal epithelium and the infiltration by some monocytes.
6. Hematoxylin bodies: pathognomonic lesions of LN. Tissue equivalent of LE cells. Structures of lilac hue, blurry edges, poorly-defined, immersed in underlying tissue, isolated or grouped, larger or smaller than a cell nucleus. Edges of hematoxylin material. It has been found in 1-2% of biopsies of LN.

Chronic lesions:

1. Segmental glomerular scars: resulting from the proliferative and necrotizing lesions.
2. Sclerotized glomeruli: in addition to scarring of active lesions, they may also occur during the evolution of class V, as a result of aging or hypertension.
3. Fibrous crescent: fibrous tissue resulting from chronic cell growth. Can be adherent to the glomerular scars.

Activity and Chronicity Indices

- Provide semiquantitative information regarding the severity of acute or chronic injury to the glomerular and tubulointerstitial compartments of the kidney. For glomerular compartment, each active and chronic item is graded as follows: 0 = absent; 1 = less than 25% of the glomeruli; 2 = 25%-50% of the glomeruli; 3 = more than 50% of the glomeruli. The most serious items, fibrinoid necrosis and crescent scores, are multiplied by a factor of 2. Tubulointerstitial items are also graded on a scale of 0 to 3: 0 = absent; 1 = mild; 2 = moderate; 3 = severe. For activity and chronicity items and scoring, see Table 4.
- The sum of these values gives a total possible activity score of 0 to 24. The total chronicity indices range from 0 to 12.

- The indices are based on the fact that active lesions are responsive to treatment, while chronic ones are not.
- Persistence of an index of similar activity, in repeated biopsies, after appropriate immunosuppressive treatment, indicates high probability of progression to renal failure.
- Poor prognosis: combination of activity index >7 and chronicity >3.
- National Institutes of Health of the United States: chronicity index >4 has a worse prognosis, and treatment is not recommended. This is disputed by other authorities.
- The ISN/RPS 2003 classification does not require the use of a formal activity or chronicity index, but incorporates elements concerning activity and chronicity.

Table 4. Activity and chronicity indices in LN

ACTIVITY INDEX (0-24)	**Score**
Cell proliferation	(0-3)
Neutrophil infiltration	(0-3)
Subendothelial hyaline deposits	(0-3)
Fibrinoid necrosis/Karyorrhexis	(0-3) x 2
Cellular crescents	(0-3) x 2
Interstitial inflammation	(0-3)
CHRONICITY INDEX (0-12)	**Score**
Glomerular sclerosis	(0-3)
Fibrous crescents	(0-3)
Tubular atrophy	(0-3)
Interstitial fibrosis	(0-3)

Case: A 24-year-old, single white female, complaining of generalized edema, hematuria, oliguria, and foamy urine. Reported hypertension of recent origin. Tests: urinalysis with +4 proteinuria, leukocyturia (20-25), hematuria (180-200), hyaline casts; proteinuria of 5.5 g/24 h; creatinine: 2.4; C3: 0.257 (normal range: 0.9-1.8); C4: 0.053 (normal range: 0.1-0.4); antinuclear antibody (ANA): reactive; albumin: 2.0 g/dL; anti-DNA antibody: 1:40.

Biopsy: GLOMEULI: endocapillary proliferation was found in all 20 glomeruli obtained from the renal biopsy; 10 glomeruli with leukocyte infiltration; 08 glomeruli with wire loop or hyaline thrombi; 02 glomeruli with crescents and one with necrosis. TUBULOINTERSTITIAL: mild interstitial fibrosis and tubular atrophy; foci of interstitial fibrosis and tubular atrophy. VESSELS: mild intimal fibrosis. IMMUNOFLUORESCENCE: strong glomerular capillary and mesangial staining for IgA, IgG, IgM, C3, kappa, lambda and C1q. DIAGNOSIS: Class IV LN. Activity index = 12/24; Chronicity Index = 2/12.

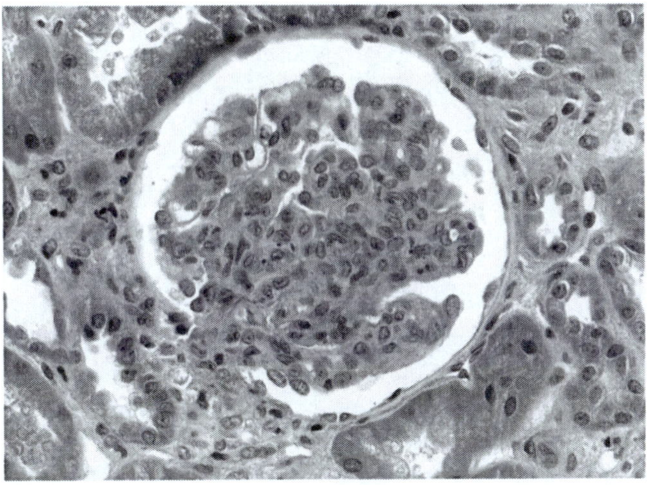

Figure 3. Masson's trichrome: intense endocapillary proliferation with occlusion of many capillary loops.

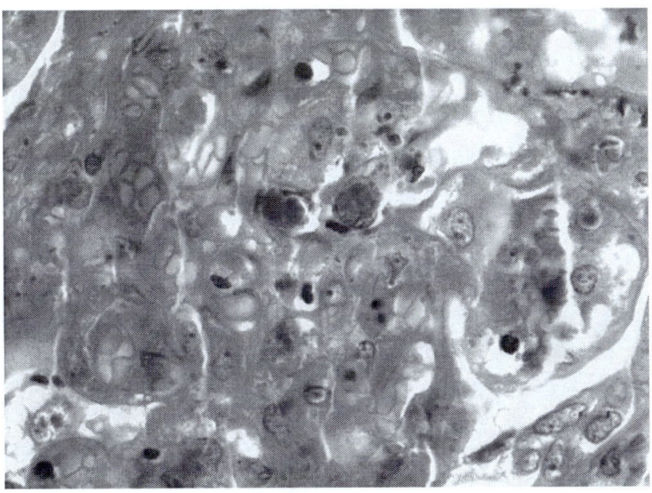

Figure 4. Hematoxylin and Eosin (H&E): showing hematoxylin corpuscles with rounded aspect, smudged, lilac, in capillary loops.

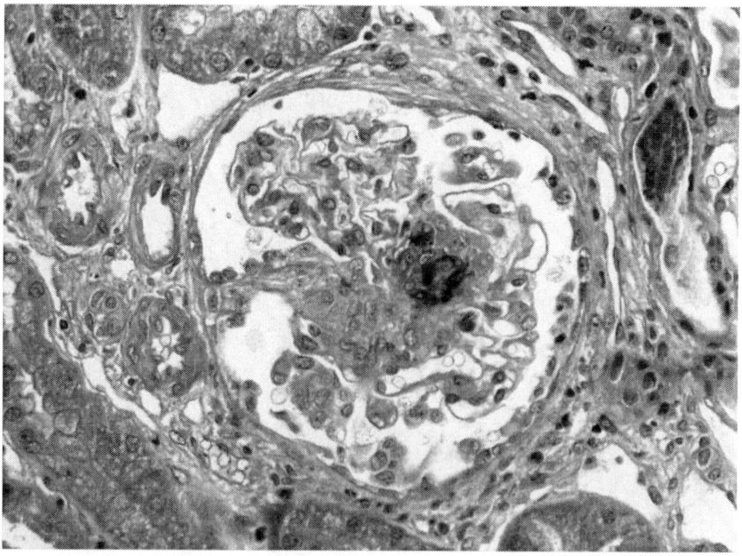

Figure 5. Masson's trichrome: necrosis in the central region of capillary tufts showing deposition of fibrin, characterized by fuchsin reactive material, in addition to formation of small crescents.

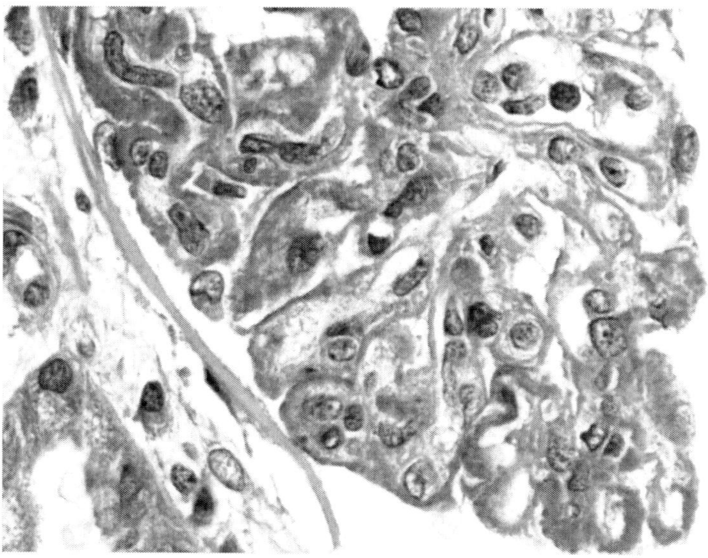

Figure 6. Masson's trichrome: massive deposition of subendothelial hyaline material (wire loop).

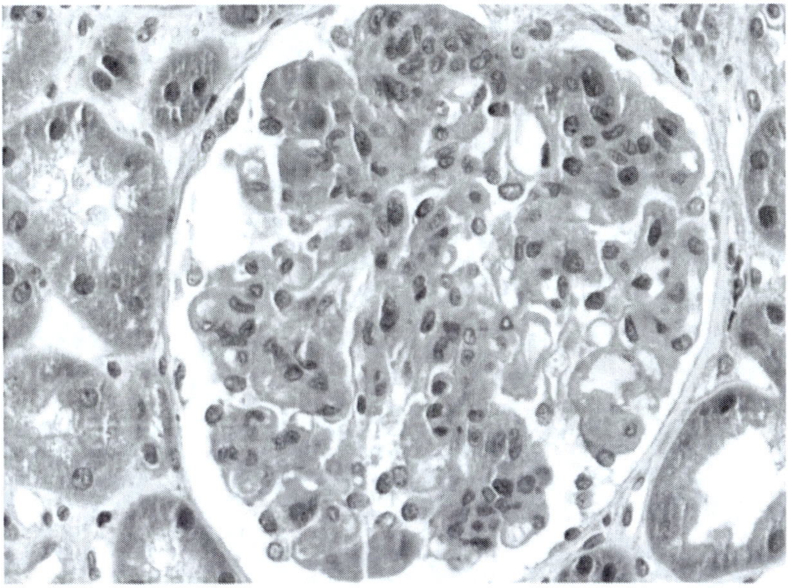

Figure 7. Masson's trichrome: deposition of hyaline material blocking the capillary lumen.

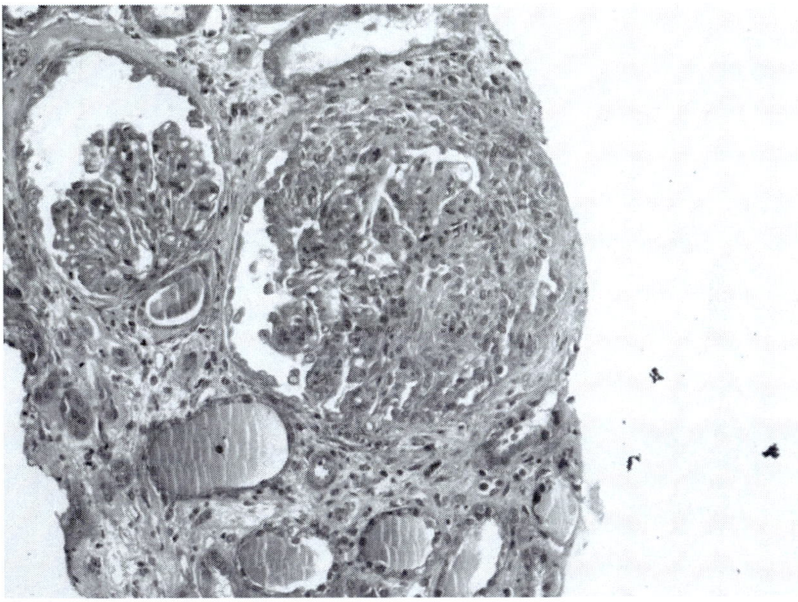

Figure 8. Masson's trichrome: showing cellular crescent involving almost the entire circumference of the glomerulus.

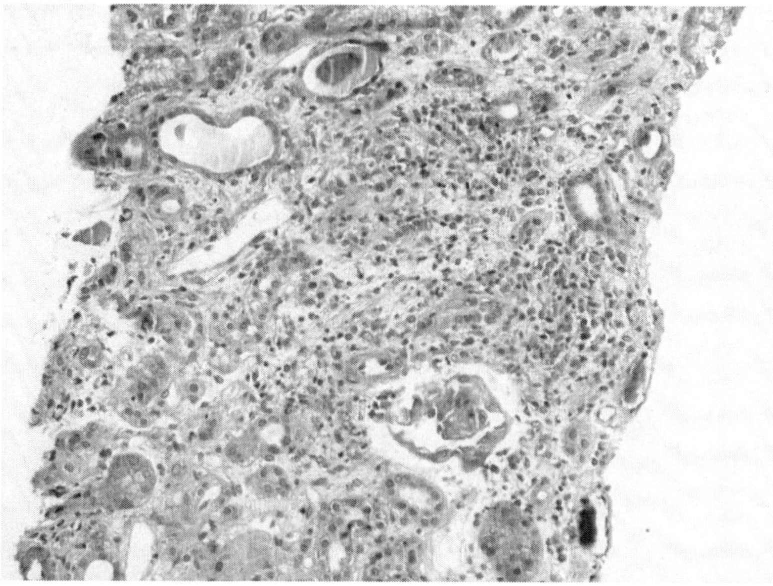

Figure 9. Masson's trichrome: chronic inflammatory infiltrate.

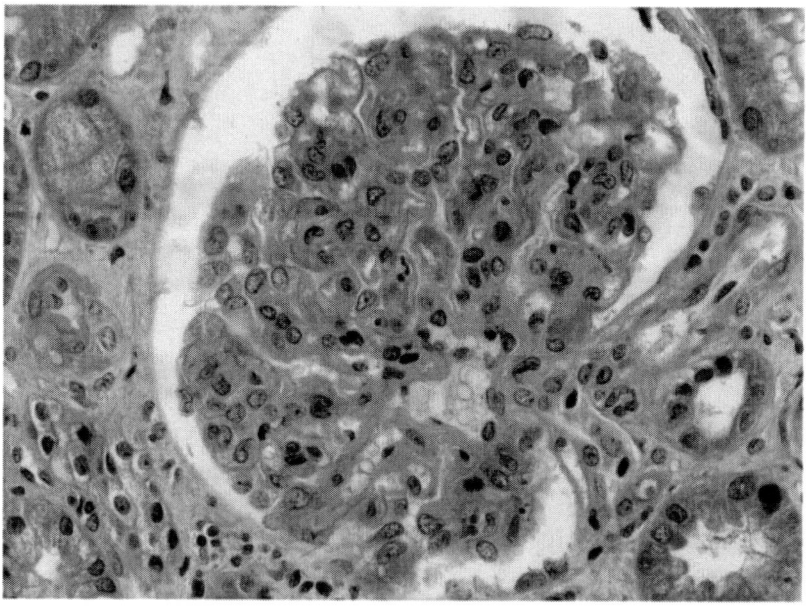

Figure 10. Masson's trichrome: glomerular acute leukocyte infiltration and endocapillary proliferation.

Histological Notes:

1) Our experience shows that the absence of "full house" staining and inconsistent positivity for C1q in patients who underwent pulse therapy is not uncommon. In these cases, it is not possible to confirm the diagnosis of LN by histology alone.
2) In any biopsy that shows "full house" staining and/or moderate to strong C1q intensity, one should consider the possibility of lupus.
3) The IF shows comma-shaped granular to pseudolinear subendothelial deposits. Usually accompanied by mesangial positivity. Epithelial deposits in more than 50% of the glomerular capillary tufts in more than 50% of the glomeruli ensure the concomitant diagnosis of class V.
4) Signs of fibrinoid necrosis: karyorrhectic debris and deposition of intensely eosinophilic fibrillar material upon H&E and fuchsin staining reactive to Masson's trichrome.

Note: the endocapillary hypercellularity results from endocapillary proliferation and leukocyte infiltration.

Differential Diagnosis:

- **Class III:** all forms of segmental and focal glomerulonephritis (NIgA, Henoch-Schönlein purpura, focal and segmental pauci-immune necrotizing glomerulonephritis, glomerulonephritis secondary to endocarditis, post-infectious glomerulonephritis).
- **Class IV:** NIgA, membranoproliferative glomerulonephritis, cryoglobulinemia, acute post-infectious glomerulonephritis, pauci-immune necrotizing glomerulonephritis.

Treatment:

- **Class III and IV:** the therapy for these two classes is based on an initial phase (or phase of induction) and a maintenance phase. The induction phase consists of a pulse with intravenous glucocorticoid for 3 days, followed by oral daily prednisone 0.5-1 mg/kg initially, reduced to the lowest effective dose within a few weeks, plus an immunosuppressive agent (cyclophosphamide or mycophenolate). In African-Americans and Hispanics, mycophenolate seems to be better.

After that, maintenance therapy with mycophenolate, in smaller doses, or azathioprine should be used.

Chapter 4

Class V

Clinical:

- The class V LN is marked by proteinuria, which can be nephrotic (60-70% of the time). Corresponding to 8-22% of the biopsies. Hematuria is found in 50% of cases and hypertension in 25%. More than 1/3 of the cases of class V present clinically without any other manifestation of SLE, and approximately 1/3 have negative autoantibodies. Renal failure is very uncommon.
- Up to one third, class V before other overt systemic manifestations of SLE.
- Class V lupus nephritis may occur in combination with classes III or IV.
- Patient with pure membranous LN experience an indolent course, similar to that of primary membranous glomerulonephritis. Renal survival of 80% in 5 years.

Morphology:

- Characterized by changes in the GBM similar to those of membranous idiopathic glomerulonephritis. The preponderant finding by LM is the homogeneous thickening of the GBM. However, morphologic lesions can differ according to the evolutionary pathologic changes occurring in GBM.
- Initially there are no detectable changes on LM. The earliest change is a "moth-eaten" appearance of the GBM seen in en face sections

stained with methenamine silver. As deposits persist, linear "spikes" protrude from the outer side of the GBM. With progressive GBM reaction, the matrix encircles the deposits resulting in a chain-like appearance. With disease progression the GBM become diffusely thickened, demonstrable with silver staining. All the changes are a result of the response of the GBM to the subepithelial deposition of immune complexes.

Case: A 27-year-old woman with history of SLE showed abnormal laboratory finding on follow up. Urinalysis: protein: +1; leukocytes absent; red blood cells (RBC) 1/high-power field (HPF); urinary protein excretion: 7.8 g/dL. Serum laboratory tests: creatinine: 0.52 mg/dL; albumin: 3.1g/dL; hemoglobin: 12 g/dL; hematocrit: 36%; white blood cells: 6.200/mL; ANA: 1:200 (speckled pattern); anti-DNA: negative; C3 and C4 was normal.

Biopsy: GLOMERULI: 14 glomeruli, all within normal limits, except for the presence of global and diffuse thickening of the GBM, with spikes on silver staining. TUBULE-INTERSTITIUM: within normal limits. BLOOD VESSELS: within normal limits. IMMUNOFLUORESCENCE: uniform granular subepithelial deposits of IgG (3+, on scale 0 to +3), C3 (3+), IgA (++), IgM (+), C1q (2+), λ (3+) and κ (2+) light chain in the capillary wall and focal deposits in the mesangium. Diagnosis: class V for LN.

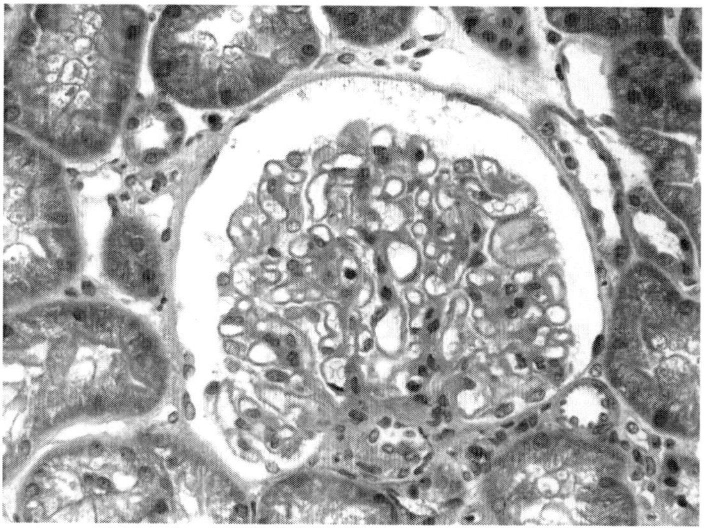

Figure 11. Masson's trichrome: Delicate thickening, global, of capillary loops, with minimal change of cellularity. Some peripheral loops, slightly "ring-like," were noted.

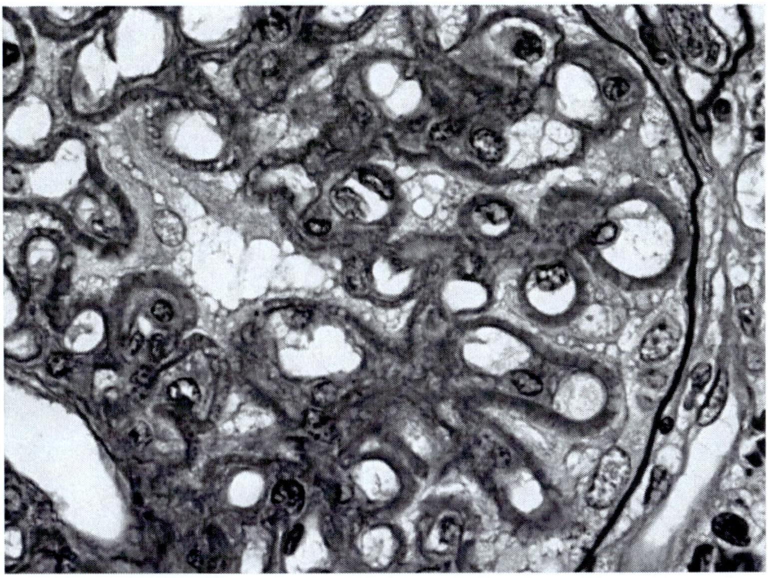

Figure 12. Periodic acid-Schiff: the "spiked" appearance in tangential sections of the GBM.

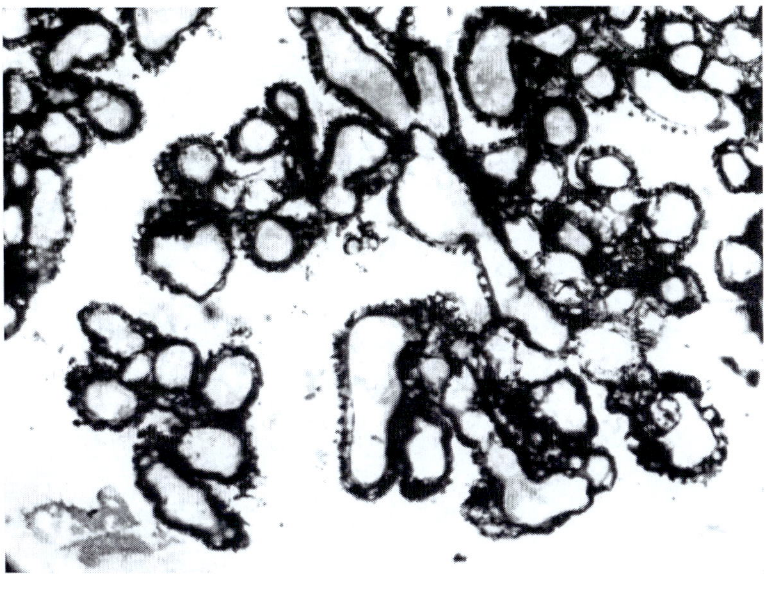

Figure 13. Jones' Methenamine Silver: the "spiked" appearance in tangential sections of the GBM.

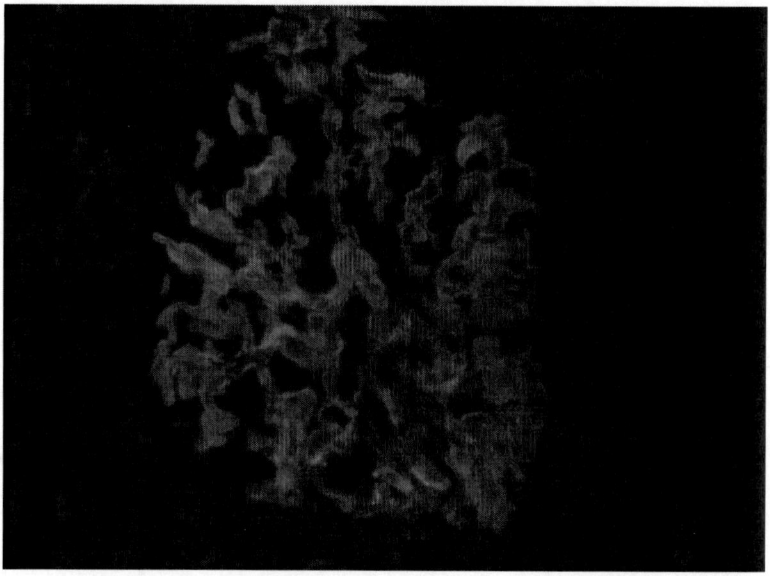

Figure 14. IgG: moderate granular capillary loop staining. Note substantial extension to mesangium (very common in secondary membranous glomerulonephritis (MGN), particularly lupus).

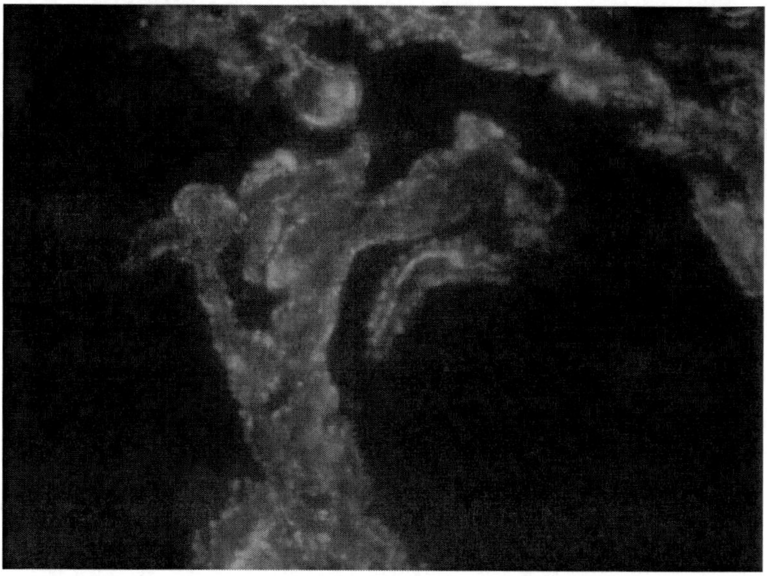

Figure 15. C1q: In class V LN, the immune deposits may occur at subepithelial, subendothelial, and mesangial sites. Positivity for IgA, IgM, and mainly C1q, is very common in membranous lupus.

Histological Notes:

1) Findings of secondary MGN: Endocapillary proliferation, increased leukocyte infiltration, IF positive for IgA, and/or IgM, and/or C1q, in addition to extension to mesangium and positivity in tubular basement membrane (TBM) and Bowman's capsule.
2) The presence of mesangial hypercellularity, without occlusion of the lumen of the capillary loop, which is seen in class II, is commonly found in Class V.
3) Presence of typical grade IV lesions, including endocapillary proliferation with closing loop, classifies the injury as class IV, as does the presence of subendothelial deposits visible on LM.
4) Subendothelial deposits (class IV) should be differentiated from those subepithelial (V). The latter are thinner granular deposits, more regular, with sharper definition and irregular outer surface.
   - A few subendothelial deposits may be found in proliferative classes. However, an additional diagnosis of membranous LN in a class III or class IV requires that more than half the glomeruli show evidence of subepithelial deposits (by LM and/or by IF) in more than half the loops.

Note: class V mixed with features of III or IV must be reported in order of the more severe (III and IV) followed by the least severe (V).

Therapeutic

- **Class V:** in patients with asymptomatic and non-nephrotic proteinuria, immunosuppressant therapy is not indicated, unless extra-renal manifestations are present. In patients with nephrotic proteinuria, therapy should be initiated with mycophenolate 2-3 g/day, plus prednisone 0.5 mg/kg/day for six months. After this, maintenance therapy consists of mycophenolate or azathioprine in reduced doses [1, 8]. In case of association with class III or IV, treatment is also determined by the most severe class.

Chapter 5

Class VI

Advanced renal Insufficiency with variable non-nephrotic proteinuria and inactive urinary sediment. Systemic hypertension is present and the serology is usually negative. More than 90% of glomeruli have global sclerosis; in some, one can notice an increase in cellularity. Marked tubular atrophy and interstitial fibrosis develop along with glomerular changes. The majority represent an advanced stage of LN.

Case: A 10-year old boy was presented to our department with a 2-month history of anasarca, gross hematuria and hypertension. Serum creatinine and albumin levels were 8.1mg/dL and 2.5g/dL, respectively. The urinary protein excretion was 1.1g/24h.

Biopsy: GLOMERULI: all 12 glomeruli showed global sclerosis associated with fibrous crescent in most. TUBULOINTERSTITIAL: advanced interstitial fibrosis and tubular atrophy with inflammatory infiltration. VESSELS: within the normal limits. IMMUNOFLUORESCENCE: intense staining for IgA, IgG, IgM, C3, Kappa, Lambda, and C1q in sclerotic glomeruli. DIAGNOSIS: Advanced chronic glomerulonephritis compatible with LN class VI.

Follow up: After renal biopsy, results of additional laboratory studies confirmed the clinical suspicion of SLE, with an antinuclear antibody titer of 1:3200 and anti–double-stranded DNA level of 26.3 IU/mL.

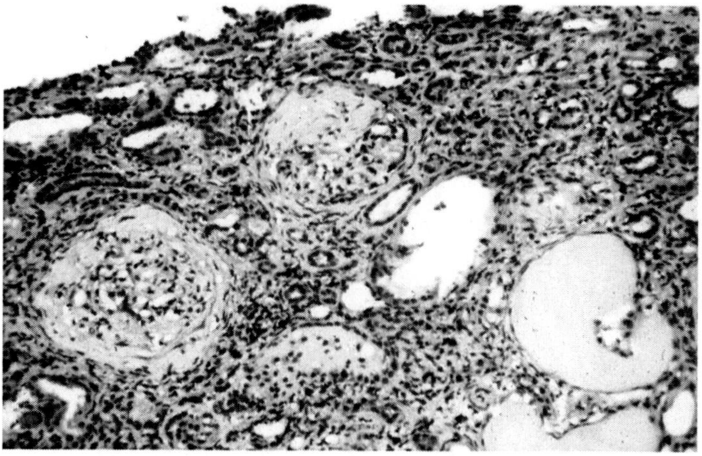

Figure 16. Hematoxylin and Eosin: class VI NL with advanced chronic changes of kidney parenchyma, including tubular atrophy, advanced interstitial fibrosis, mononuclear inflammation, and global glomerulosclerosis.

Chapter 6

Tubulointerstitial Lesions

- Tubulointerstitial disease of the kidneys is a well-recognized feature of LN, occurring in 66% of kidney biopsy specimens of patients with SLE.
- Tubulointerstitial disease may progress independent of glomerular disease in some patients.
- Injury in the tubulointerstitial compartment can be found in all classes of lupus; however, it is more common in proliferative classes, mainly in class IV. The following tubular changes can be found: droplets of reabsorption of cytoplasmic proteins and lipid vacuoles in proximal tubules of patients with significant proteinuria; acute tubular necrosis in proliferative classes or very high proteinuria; and hematic casts in proliferative classes.
- Immune deposits may be found in TBM, interstitial capillary walls, and/or interstitial collagen.

Tubulointerstitial Nephritis in Lupus

- Clinically characterized by renal dysfunction, minimal leukocyturia and hematuria, and proteinuria less than 1 g/24 h.
- Edema and interstitial inflammation are frequent findings in serious proliferative nephritis, usually accompanied by IgG deposits within the TBM, peritubular capillaries, and interstitial collagen. Infiltration is mainly by mononuclear cells: lymphocytes, monocytes, and plasma

cells. The presence of tubulointerstitial nephritis in classes II and V is not common.

- The predominant or isolated presence of tubulointerstitial changes in the setting of minimal or absent glomerular abnormalities in patients with SLE is very rare. To the best of our knowledge, only twelve cases have been reported.
- Pathogenesis: circulating immune complexes specifically interacting with tubulointerstitial autoantigens.
- Treatment: often there is a good response to corticosteroids.

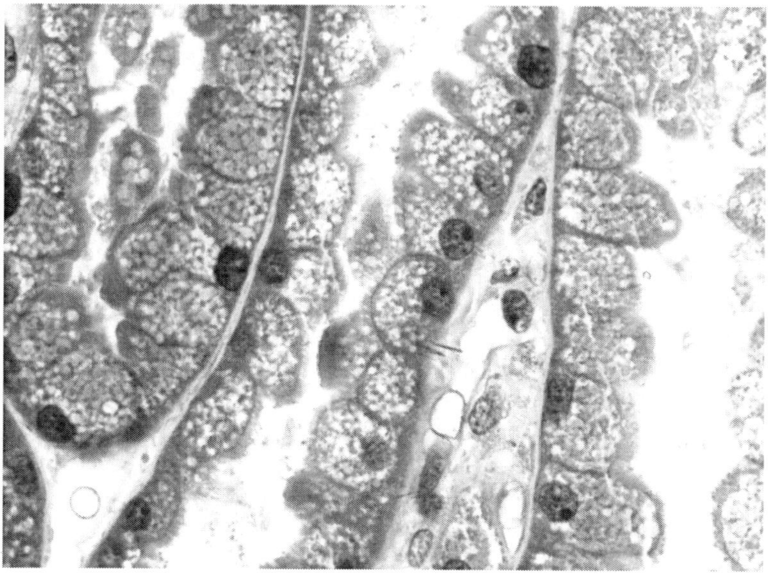

Figure 17. Tubular epithelial cells with clear lipid and hyaline protein droplets.

Case: A 52-year-old woman with a 10-year history of SLE. Serum creatinine level was 1.4 mg/dL and urinalysis at the time showed 3+ protein, 3+ blood, and red blood cell casts. Serum C3 level of 52 mg/dL (normal range, 80 to 170 mg/dL); and C4 level of 14 mg/dL (normal range, 16 to 40 mg/dL).

Renal Biopsy: GLOMERULI: 15 glomeruli in the biopsy sample, of which 13 exhibited global proliferation; two with leucocyte infiltration; one with global sclerosis; and 4 exhibited crescent formation. TUBULOINTERSTITIUM: some areas with dense lymphocytic infiltrate; mild interstitial fibrosis. VESSELS: IMMUNOFLUORESCENCE: granular positivity along the GBM and mesangium for IgG (3+, on 0–3 scale), IgA

(3+), IgM (1+), C3 (3+), C1q (2+), Kappa (3+), and Lambda (3+); positive staining for IgG and C3 along the renal tubular basement membrane. DIAGNOSIS: Class IV LN with significant interstitial inflammation component.

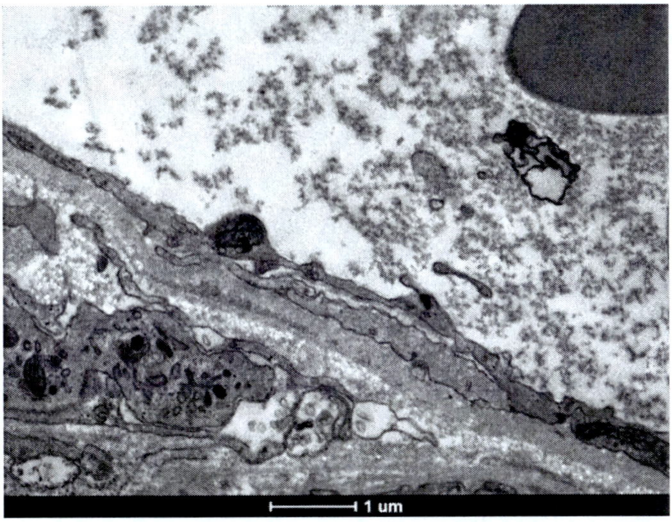

Figure 18. Electron Microscopy: tubular basement membrane electron-dense deposits.

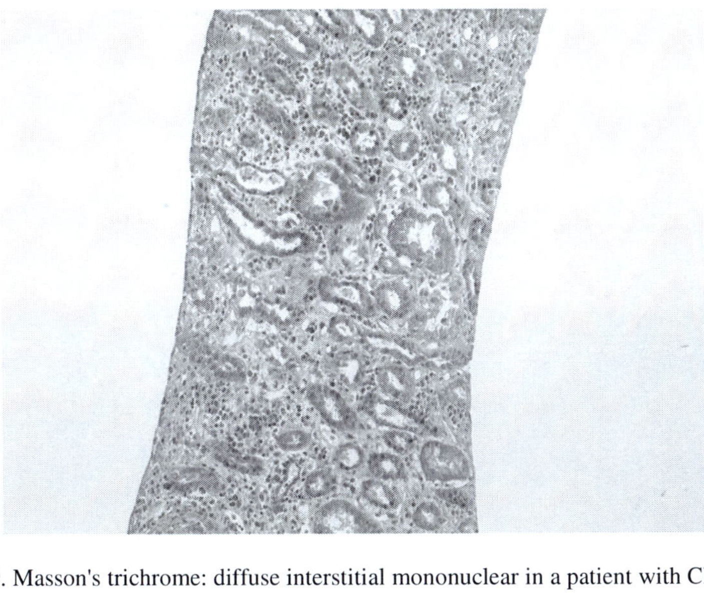

Figure 19. Masson's trichrome: diffuse interstitial mononuclear in a patient with Class IV LN.

Rhabdomyolysis

- Rhabdomyolysis is a rare condition in immunological diseases, including those that occur concomitantly with myositis.
- Seven cases of rhabdomyolysis have been described in the literature: 2 had discoid lupus and 5 SLE.
- In some patients, the precipitating factors responsible for the induction of rhabdomyolysis were identified. The use of myotoxic drugs in one case and infection (bacterial and viral) in three cases. In the remaining cases, precipitating factors were not identified.
- Treatment is performed with carefully monitored hydration.

Case: A patient with a history of lupus for 13 years developed intense muscle pain, which led to limiting mild activities (e.g., getting up from a chair), with a sudden increase in creatinine levels, mild proteinuria, and without microscopic hematuria. Muscle biopsy showed necrosis and regeneration, with mild inflammatory infiltrate.

Biopsy: GLOMERULI: within normal limits. TUBULOINTERSTITIUM: dilated tubules with foci of epithelial cellular necrosis. VESSEL: mild fibrous intimal thickening. IMMUNOFLUORESCENCE: negative.

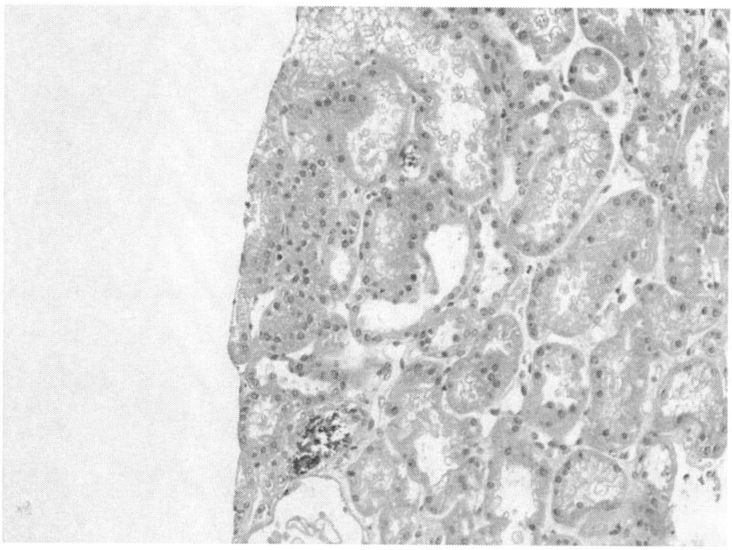

Figure 20. Masson's trichrome: changes of acute tubular necrosis (tubular dilation, planing, and epithelial desquamation), associated with the presence of reddish granular casts.

Chapter 7

Vascular Lesions

- Although these lesions influence prognosis, they are not considered in the classifications, nor are the activity and chronicity indices. For this reason, they are easily overlooked by the pathologist. Note: the presence of vascular injury should also be ruled out by IF fragment analysis.

1. Arteriosclerosis and arteriolosclerosis: not specific to lupus, common in patients with a history of chronic LN of any class. Associated with aging, hypertension, immunosuppressive drugs, and is a relevant prognostic factor.

2. Non-complicated immune deposition: characteristic of classes III and IV, but can occur in II and V. It occurs mainly in small arteries and arterioles. On IF, the vascular deposits have "full house" staining and positivity for C1q. They have no clinical effect or prognostic implications. The majority of cases are not detected by LM, and cases with deposits of this intensity are very rare. It is highly characteristic of LN. Unlike hyaline arteriolosclerosis, deposition occurs mainly in the subendothelial region.

Case: A 29 year-old female patient, with joint pain for 5 years, treated as "rheumatism." About 5 months prior, she noticed dark and foamy urine. The examination showed violaceous nodules in the lower limbs, and malar erythema. Laboratory tests: HB: 7.4 g/dL; ANA (speckled >1: 800); C3 low, antineutrophil cytoplasmic antibodies (ANCA) was not reactive. Urinalysis: leukocytes 4-6, red blood cells 2-3, waxy and granular casts, protein +3.

Biopsy: GLOMERULI: 13 glomeruli, all within normal limits, except for the presence of mild to moderate hypercellularity. TUBULE-INTERSTITIUM: mild interstitial fibrosis and tubular atrophy; rare foci of chronic inflammatory infiltrate. BLOOD VESSELS: within normal limits. IMMUNOFLUORESCENCE: moderate positivity in mesangium, global and diffuse, with anti-IgG, C3, and C1q antibodies. Immunoglobulins and complement fractions were also observed in vessels. Diagnosis: LN class II and vasculopathy with deposition of immune complexes.

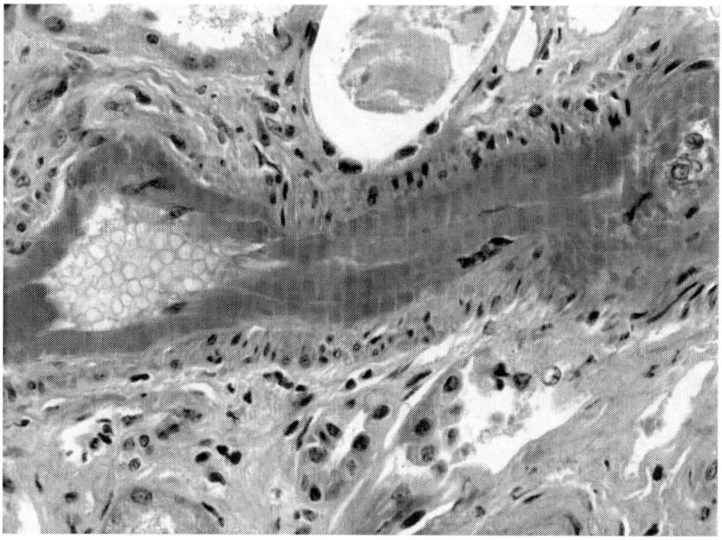

Figure 21. Masson's trichrome: showing massive subendothelial hyaline deposits, with reduction of the lumen.

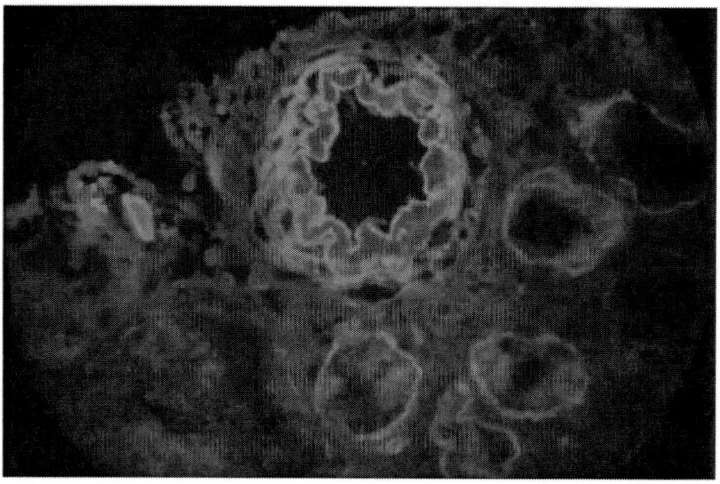

Figure 22. C1q: showing intense subendothelial staining in the vessels.

3. Non-inflammatory necrotizing vasculopathy: Associated with class IV, and affects primarily arterioles. This term is used for cases of necrotizing, non-inflammatory vascular lesions. The hallmark is deposition of fibrinoid material expanding the intima and occluding the vascular lumen. Myocyte and endothelium necrosis can occur. There is no inflammatory infiltration. On IF, deposits of IgG and fibrin indicate the combination of immune complex deposits and intravascular coagulation. Clinical picture is severe hypertension and renal failure with rapid progression. The prognosis is poor.

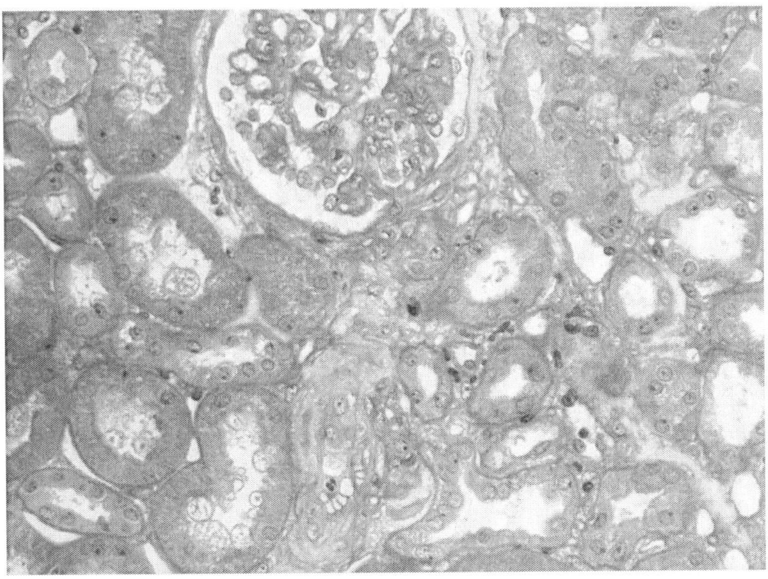

Figure 23. Masson's trichrome: the lumen of an arteriole sharply reduced by deposits of reddish material strongly suggestive of fibrin.

4. Necrotizing Arteritis: rare Injury in LN. It may be isolated or associated with systemic vasculitis. Histologically, necrotizing arteritis is characterized by fibrinoid necrosis and leukocyte infiltration of the vascular wall. It occurs in any class, regardless of glomerular activity.

5. Thrombotic Microangiopathy (TMA): affects small arteries, arterioles, and glomerular capillaries. TMA can occur in several different scenarios, such as the antiphospholipid antibody syndrome, lupus anticoagulant syndrome, hemolytic-uremic syndrome, thrombotic thrombocytopenic purpura, syndrome overlaps with scleroderma, malignant hypertension, use of calcineurin inhibitors, etc. It can also occur in any classes of LN, or it can be an isolated finding. Histologically presents with thrombi in glomerular capillaries, small arteries and arterioles, enlargement of the subendothelial region, mesangiolysis, mucoid degeneration of the intima, and fragments of erythrocytes in thrombus if deposition of fibrin is shown, without associated immune complexes. Laboratory tests can be positive for lupus anticoagulant, antiphospholipid antibody, and autoantibody to von Willebrand factor cleaving protease.

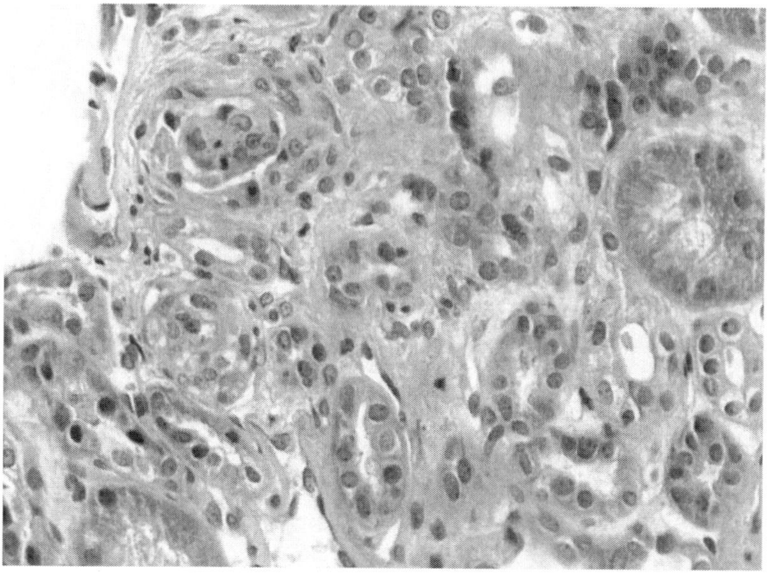

Figure 24. Masson's trichrome: another arteriole in the same case, showing myocyte necrosis.

Case: A 14-year-old patient, female, with generalized edema a month prior. The patient also had seizures. Laboratory tests: creatinine 3.4 mg/dL; direct Coombs was positive (3 samples); ANA: 1/400; anti-DNA: 1/20; C3: 0.65 g/dL (normal range, 0.9-1.8 g/dL), C4: 0.065 g/dL (normal range, 0.1-0.4 g/dL).

Biopsy: GLOMERULI: All 17 glomeruli in the biopsy specimen show moderate to marked proliferation and partial occlusion of capillary loops; 9 with thrombi in the vascular pole and signs of secondary ischemia. TUBULE-INTERSTITIUM: foci of mild interstitial fibrosis and tubular atrophy. BLOOD VESSELS: within normal limits, except for the changes described above in glomerular vascular pole. IMMUNOFLUORESCENCE: diffuse and global IgG, IgA, IgM, C3, kappa, lambda and C1q positivity in mesangium and GBM. Fibrinogen was observed in the glomerular vascular pole. Diagnosis: Thrombotic microangiopathy and LN class IV.

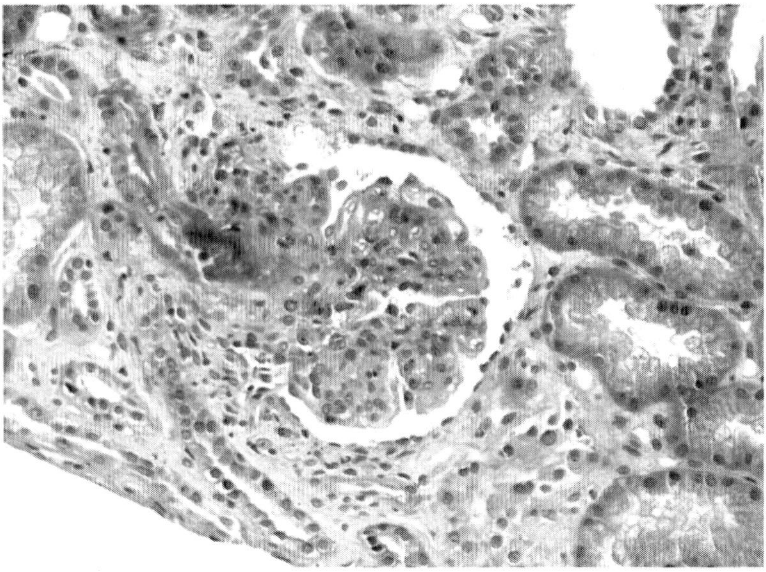

Figure 25. Masson's trichrome: a thrombus in the arteriole extended to the glomerular vascular pole.

Antiphospholipid Antibody Syndrome (APS)

- Defined by the occurrence of two or more thrombotic episodes or abortion in patients with serological evidence of antiphospholipid antibody, which can be lupus anticoagulant or anticardiolipin antibodies.
- Divided into primary and secondary (autoimmune diseases, cancer, and infections). Among the secondary types, lupus stands out.
- Occurs in patients with both complete and incomplete criteria for lupus.
- Multisystem involvement: skin, heart, liver, lungs, brain, eyes, and kidneys. Renal involvement occurs in 6-26% of cases.
- Renal vein and artery thrombosis can occur, leading to renal infarctions and abdominal pain.

- Nephropathy caused by APS leads to hypertension (93%), chronic renal failure (87%), variable degrees of proteinuria (75%), and hematuria (56%).
- Morphologically, two patterns are found: 1) TMA - thrombi in glomeruli, arterioles, and arteries; 2) Nephropathy of antiphospholipid antibody - fibrous intimal hyperplasia, and arterial and arteriolar fibrous and fibrocellular occlusions.

Case: A young patient with SLE, on a background of hematuria and non-nephrotic proteinuria, severe hypertension, and renal failure. The assessment of antiphospholipid antibodies showed positivity for lupus anticoagulant, anticardiolipin IgM, and IgG.

Biopsy: GLOMERULI: 13 glomeruli, of which 3 were globally sclerotic. The remaining glomeruli showed ischemic collapse without proliferative changes. TUBULOINTERSTITIUM: mild to moderate focal interstitial fibrosis and tubular atrophy. VESSELS: chronic vascular lesions such as fibrous intimal hyperplasia of arterioles. IMMUNOFLUORESCENCE: mild mesangial staining with IgA, IgM, IgG e C3. DIAGNOSIS: Nephropathy of antiphospholipid antibody secondary to SLE.

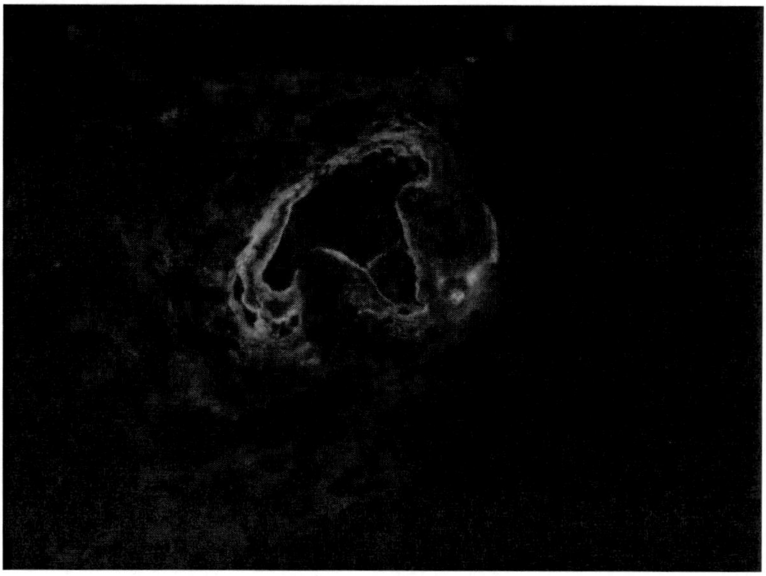

Figure 26. Fibrinogen: fibrin deposition in vascular walls (vessel in transverse section).

Catastrophic Antiphospholipid Antibody Syndrome (CAPS)

- In a small number of cases, there is an acute disseminated syndrome, with multiple vascular occlusions, associated with the presence of antiphospholipid antibodies.
- Most cases present with renal dysfunction, cerebrovascular disease, myocardial infarction, and hypertension. The majority of patients reported a history of mild or inactive SLE.
- Renal involvement in CAPS is much more frequent than usual APS, 78% of cases.
- The anticardiolipin IgG titers are elevated, and the lupus anticoagulant is positive. A precipitating event, such as a viral infection, use of medication, or the postpartum period, may be present in some cases. CAPS is fatal in 40% of cases.

Chapter 8

Lupus Overlap Diseases

Overlap Syndrome

- Defined by overlapping characteristics of SLE and other rheumatological diseases (scleroderma and polymyositis). Also called mixed connective tissue disease.
- The diagnosis depends on the presence of autoantibodies against extractable nuclear antigens (anti-ENA; also called RNP) greater than 1:600, and at least three of the following characteristic: hand edema, synovitis, myositis, Raynaud's phenomenon, and acrosclerosis. Recently, two more specific antibodies were described: U1-snRNP and hnRNP-A2.
- Renal involvement was less frequent and often less severe than in SLE. It is usually more common in children (33-50%) than in adults (10-26%).
- Renal manifestations are quite variable. Approximately 20% have mild proteinuria, with or without microscopic hematuria. One third of cases show intense proteinuria, with or without the full nephrotic syndrome. A few patients have typical changes of involvement by scleroderma: severe hypertension, thrombotic microangiopathy, and acute renal failure.
- Two histological findings are described: 1) immune complex glomerulonephritis, which resemble the patterns found in SLE and 2) the vascular lesions are similar to those in scleroderma. In the glomerulus: membranous nephropathy (35-40%), mesangial lesions

(35%), membranoproliferative (7%), mesangial proliferative (7%), amyloidosis, minimal change disease, and crescentic glomerulonephritis. In vessels (small and medium): mucoid degeneration or intimal sclerosis (most common), hyperplasia of the media, and, more rarely, fibrinoid necrosis and myocardial infarction.

Case: A 48-year-old woman with progressive dyspnea, arthralgia, Raynaud phenomena, and myalgia for two years. A urinalysis showed 3+ protein, a hematuria of 50-60/HPF, and a leukocyturia of 40-50/HPF. A 24-hour urine collection revealed 1.1 g of protein. FAN, anti-SM and anti-RNP were positives and anti-DNA negative.

Biopsy: GLOMERULI: 9 glomeruli show only mild mesangial hypercellularity. TUBULOINTERSTITIAL: focal mild interstitial fibrosis. VESSELS: arterioles with "onion skin" concentric appearance. IMMUNOFLUORESCE: diffuse moderate mesangial staining for IgA, IgG, IgM, C3, kappa, lambda, C1q. DIAGNOSIS: Class II LN and sclerodema (overlap syndrome).

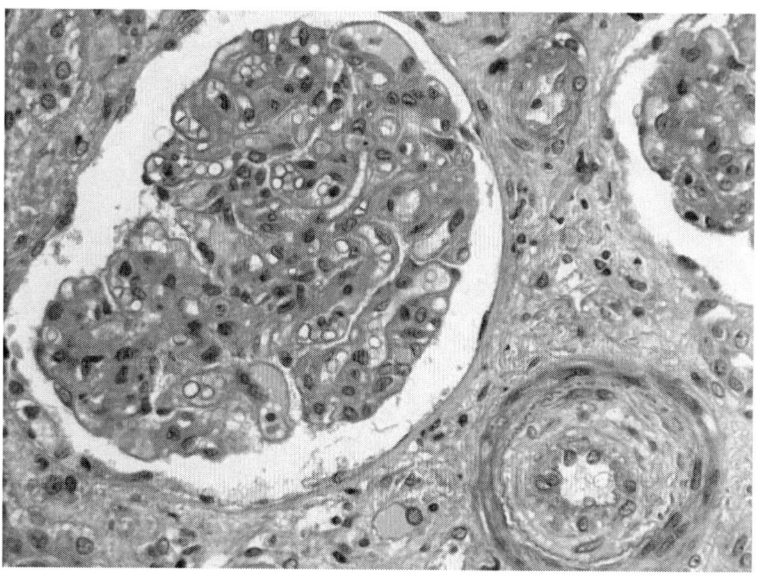

Figure 27. Masson's trichrome: glomeruli with mild mesangial hypercellularity and arteriole with hyperplastic arteriolosclerosis in a patient with overlap syndrome (SLE + scleroderma).

Lupus and HIV

- Although the most common form of glomerular injury in HIV-positive patients is the collapsing form of segmental glomerulosclerosis, some patients manifest a clinical and histological picture of lupus.
- The pathogenesis is not completely understood. Possibilities: direct action of the virus, alteration of the immune system, or drug toxicity.
- In addition to the renal lesion, HIV infection shares other features with SLE: anemia, leukopenia, multi-organ involvement, serositis, and renal disease.
- Unlike LN, lupus associated with HIV primarily affects black men or children with perinatal infection caused by HIV.
- Kidney disease presents with: hematuria, proteinuria, nephrotic syndrome, and renal failure.
- The biopsy can reveal any existing class in LN (II, III, IV, V, III + V). Sometimes overlapping with a collapsing form may be present.
- Together with SLE, concomitant vascular lesions, such as thrombotic microangiopathy and necrotizing arteritis, have been reported.

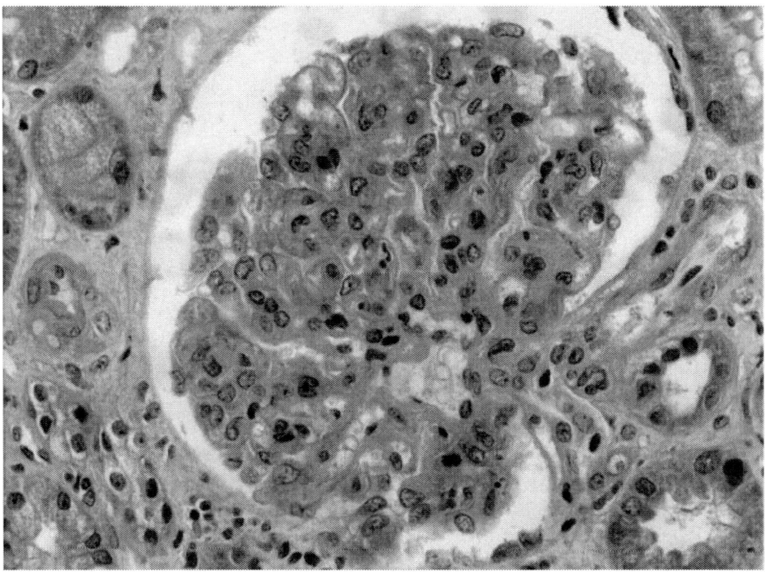

Figure 28. Masson's trichrome: Proliferation, infiltration and deposits in a patient with class IV LN secondary to HIV.

Case: A 45-year-old white woman was diagnosed with HIV infection and followed up for 10 years. She was admitted in our hospital with face and lower limbs edema, gross hematuria, and asthenia. Serum laboratory exams showed: proteinuria 6g/24h; serum albumin 1.6 mg/dL; serum creatinine level 1.0 mg/dL. Urinalysis revealed hematuria and leukocyturia. Anti-nuclear antibodies were negative and C3 was normal.

Biopsy: GLOMERULI: endocapillary proliferation in all 12 glomeruli available in the kidney biopsy; 05 with leukocyte infiltration; 05 with subendothelial deposits; 02 with crescent. TUBULOINTERSTITIUM: mild to moderate diffuse interstitial fibrosis and tubular atrophy. VESSELS: moderate interstitial fibrosis. IMMUNOFLUORESCE: IgA (+2), IgG (+2), IgM (+), C3 (++), kappa (2+), lambda (2+) and C1q (2+).

Anca-Associated Nephritis

- It should be suspected in any patient with LN associated with necrosis and crescents, but without prominent proliferation of endocapillary and subendothelial deposits.
- ANCA react with components of cytoplasmic granules in neutrophils that express myeloperoxidase (MPO) or proteinase 3 (PR3).
- We do not know if ANCA are the result of autoimmunity in lupus, or a stand-alone process. In fact, the incidence of ANCA in SLE ranges from 15-20%. On the other hand, patients with acute renal failure due to pauci-immune necrotizing and crescentic glomerulonephritis with ANCA seropositivity can present with positive lupus serologies.
- ANCA-associated nephritis can also occur in drug-induced lupus.
- Treatment: plasmapheresis and immunosuppressive therapy.

Crescentic Glomerulonephritis in Lupus

- Crescentic glomerulonephritis refers to the presence of crescents in >50% of glomeruli available in a kidney sample. According the pattern on the IF, crescentic glomerulonephritis is classified into 3 types: pauci-immune (negative IF), mediated by immune complexes (granular pattern), and anti-GBM (linear pattern).

- Lupus is a secondary disease most commonly associated with crescentic glomerulonephritis, and is also the most common among those mediated by immune complexes. Crescents can be seen in 56.5% of the biopsies in class III and IV, and generally affect more than 50% of the glomeruli in 12.9%. This last condition is more common in class IV LN.
- The treatment is with high doses of steroids and cytotoxic drugs, as well as in other crescentic glomerulonephritis.
- Regarding patients with class IV, but with less than or equal to 50% of the glomeruli having crescents, patients with lupus crescentic glomerulonephritis have: more acute onset, severe renal manifestations, less extra-renal involvement, lower serologic activity, more glomerular necrosis, tubular atrophy, interstitial fibrosis, leukocyte infiltration, less deposition of glomerular immune complexes, worse response to treatment, and worse renal survival.

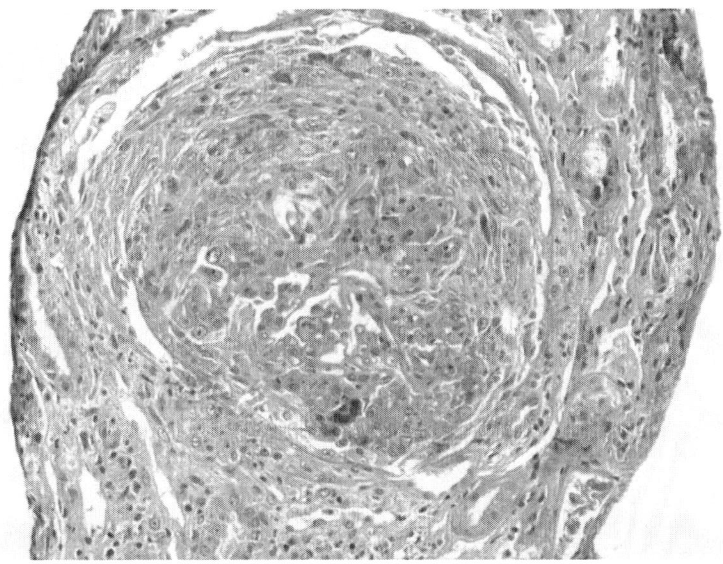

Figure 29. Masson's trichrome: cellular crescent with focal glomerular tuft necrosis in a glomerular without endocapilar proliferation.

Case: A 36 year-old woman with SLE without kidney disease. She was admitted in our service for anasarca, gross hematuria, progressive dyspnea, oliguria, and fever. Laboratory exams at admission: creatinine 8.4 mg/dL. Urinalysis: protein +2; leukocytes 50-40 cells/PHF; numerous red blood cells.

Biopsy: GLOMERULI: all 08 glomeruli with cellular crescent and without prominent hypercellularity; 05 with focal glomerular tuft necrosis. TUBULOINTERSTITIAL: moderate to severe interstitial fibrosis and tubular atrophy. VESSELS: within normal limits. IMMUNOFLUORESCENCE: sparse weak granular for IgG and C3.

Diabetes Mellitus and Lupus

- The exact prevalence of diabetes mellitus in patients who use corticosteroids therapy is unknown, but is underestimated (1.5-47%).
- The combination of SLE and DM is uncommon and can be associated with longer steroid use (especially a higher cumulative dose).

Chapter 9

Other Glomerular Lesions

Podocytopathies

Podocytopathies should be suspected in lupus patients with marked nephrotic syndrome with abrupt onset; renal biopsy with minimal or no hypercellularity, in addition to diffuse foot process effacement, and without electron-dense deposits in the GBM. A striking feature of this entity is the prompt response to treatment with immunosuppressive drugs. It has been debated whether this entity is related to a type of mesangial lupus, or if it is a fortuitous finding. The concomitant occurrence of renal injury and the onset of clinical signs of SLE strengthen the former hypothesis. Another factor is the high activity of systemic cytokines of SLE in these patients.

Case: A 41-year-old woman complaining of generalized edema and mild arthralgia for 5 months. She had proteinuria of 6-g/24 h, accompanied by leucocyturia (15-20 RBCs per high-power field). Serum creatinine was 1 mg/dL, albumin 1 g/dL, and cholesterol 420 mg/dL. Serology was positive for ANA (1:400), and negative for anti-DNA and anti-Sm.

Biopsy: GLOMERULI: 36 glomeruli, 9 of them with minimal hypercellularity. On EM, diffuse foot process effacement was seen and no electron-dense deposits was found. TUBULOINTERSTITIUM: within normal limits. BLOOD VESSELS: within normal limits. IMMUNOFLUORE-SCENCE: low positivity in mesangium, global and diffuse, with anti-IgG, IgA, IgM, C3, and C1q antibody. Diagnosis: LN class II and lupus podocytopathy, histologically similar to minimal lesion disease.

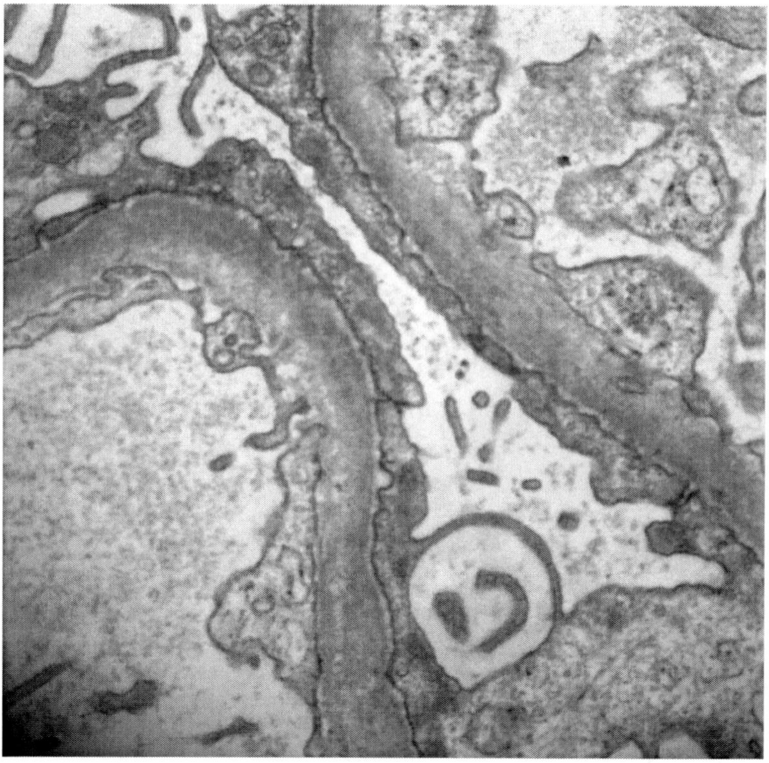

Figure 30. Electron Microscopy: foot process effacement (arrows), and absence of subendothelial and subepithelial deposits.

Amyloidosis

- Like most chronic inflammatory diseases, secondary amyloidosis (AA) has been reported in patients with SLE. However, these have become very rare, probably due to advances in the treatment of SLE.
- Serum amyloid A protein levels were significantly higher in SLE patients.
- Inherited, infectious, and inflammatory bowel diseases, which are known to cause AA amyloidosis, should be ruled out.

IgA Nephropathy and Other Glomerulopathies

- Excluding podocytopathies and amyloidosis, other glomerulopathies are rare. IgA nephropathy is the most common of these conditions.
- Based on the relative frequency of both conditions, the coexistence of primary NIgA and SLE can be an occasional finding. Both conditions are characterized by the disorders of immune function, the presence of immune complexes, and the circulating anti-C1q antibodies, besides the involvement of genetic and environmental risk factors.
- The majority of the cases described with this association reveal normal serum complement levels.
- Immunohistological findings of NIgA include glomerular mesangial deposits of IgA usually accompanied by C3 and sometimes by IgG and IgM. LN is characterized by glomerular, vascular, and tubulointerstitial lesions, with deposition of all immunoglobulins ("full house" pattern), predominantly IgG, together with C1q, C3, and C4 complement fractions.

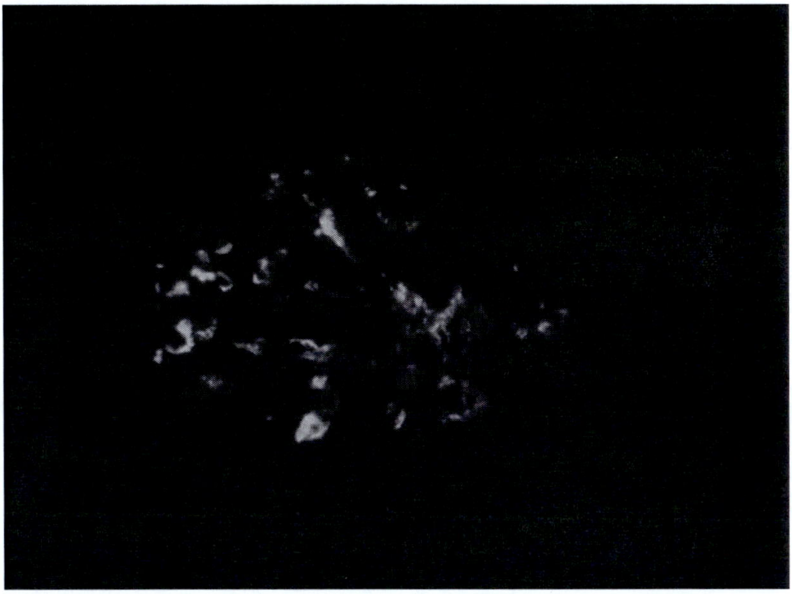

Figure 31. IgA: Glomerulus with intense global mesangial staining with antisera for IgA.

Case: A 44-year-old woman diagnosed with lupus six months previously (fever, malar rash, photosensitivity, and oral ulcers). During the assessment presented with hematuria (15-20 RBCs per high-power field) and proteinuria (3 g/ 24 h). Positive ANA (1:800), anti-DNA non-reactive, and normal complement levels.

Biopsy: GLOMERULI: 12 with only mild hypercellularity. TUBULE-INTERSTITIUM: within normal limits. BLOOD VESSELS: within normal limits. IMMUNOFLUORESCENCE: IgA (+3) and C3 (+2) in a diffuse and global mesangial pattern. Diagnosis: primary IgA nephropathy.

Chapter 10

Lupus and Drugs

Drug-Induced Lupus

- Diagnosis of drug-induced lupus is based on 3 criteria: 1) absence of lupus before drug administration; 2) ANA develops during treatment, with at least one clinical feature of SLE; 3) clinical and laboratory improvement after interruption of treatment.
- A host of drugs have been reported to cause lupus-like syndrome, including procainamide, hydralazine, isoniazid, methyldopa, and chlorpromazine.
- Renal involvement is less frequent in drug-induced lupus than in SLE.
- The histological pattern most commonly found is proliferative (focal or diffuse). Sometimes crescentic glomerulonephritis can also be found, including a necrotizing form associated with ANCA.

Nephrotoxicity Due to Treatment with Chloroquine

- Also called chloroquine-induced phospholipidosis.
- Is clinically characterized by mild proteinuria, hematuria, and renal dysfunction. The disease is reversible after withdrawal of the drug.
- May be accompanied by cardiomyopathy, proximal myopathy, keratopathy, retinopathy, and hearing loss.

- LM shows vacuolization of the podocyte cytoplasm, which had lamellar (myelin or zebra bodies) structures under electronmicroscopic observation. In the past, "myelin" bodies were described as pathognomonic of Fabry disease, but in addition to toxicity due to chloroquine, they also appear in nephropathy caused by silica, gentamicin and amiodarone.
- Patients with chloroquine-induced phospholipidosis have the same "myelin" deposits in biopsies of skeletal muscle.

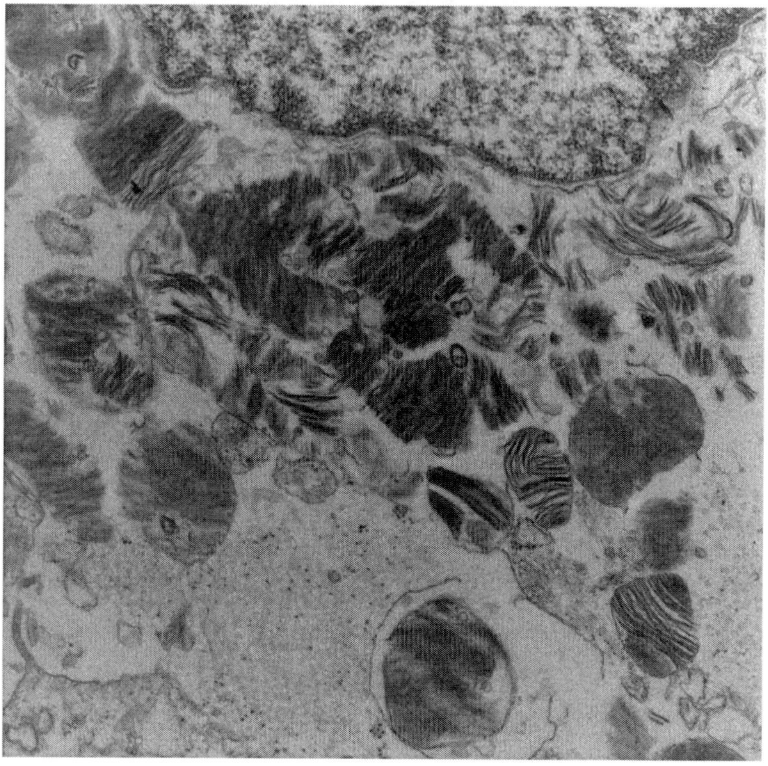

Figure 32. Electron Microscopy: laminated intra-cytoplasmic inclusions ('zebra bodies') within podocytes.

Case: A 56-year-old woman reports having SLE for about 10 years, without renal involvement, under treatment with prednisone and chloroquine since then, currently with active renal disease, and requiring biopsy for guidance of therapy.

Biopsy: GLOMERULI: all glomeruli showed only large podocytes with vacuolated cytoplasm. TUBULE-INTERSTITIUM: within normal limits. BLOOD VESSELS: within normal limits. IMMUNOFLUORESCENCE: negative. Electron Microscopy: zebra bodies inclusions within podocytes. Diagnosis: nephrotoxicity due to chloroquine.

References

Albay D, Adler SG, Philipose J, Calescibetta CC, Romansky SG, Cohen AH. Chloroquine-induced lipidosis mimicking Fabry disease. *Mod Pathol.* 2005;18:733-8.

Alarcon-Segovia D, Cardiel MH. Comparison between 3 diagnostic criteria for mixed connective tissue disease. Study of 593 patients. *J Rheumatol.* 1989;16:328

Aringer M, Smolen JS. Mixed connective tissue disease: what is behind the curtain? *Best Pract Res Clin Rheumatol.* 2007 Dec; 21:1037-49.

Banks DE, Milutinovic J, Desnick RJ, Grabowski GA, Lapp NL, Boehlecke BA. Silicon nephropathy mimicking Fabry's disease. *Am J Nephrol.* 1983 Sep-Oct;3:279-84.

Bennett R. Mixed connective tissue disease. In: Grishman E, Churg J, Needle MA, Venkataseshan VS, eds. The Kidney in Collagen Vascular Diseases. New York: Raven Press, 1993:167.

Bhargava A, Ortega LM, Nayer A, Burguera V, Jasnosz K. Necrotizing crescentic glomerulonephritis in a patient with positive serologies for lupus and antineutrophil cytoplasmic antibodies. *Nefrologia.* 2014 Sep 26;34:678-81.

Carvalho JF, Mota LM, Bonfa E. Fatal rhabdomyolysis in systemic lupus erythematosus. *Rheumatol Int.* 2010;31:1243-5.

Chen S, Tang Z, Zhang Y, Liu Z, Zhang H, Hu W, Liu Z. Significance of histological crescent formation in patients with diffuse proliferative lupus nephritis. *Am J Nephrol.* 2013;38:445-52.

Cohen SD, Kimmel PL. Immune complex renal disease and human immunodeficiency virus infection. *Semin Nephrol.* 2008;28:535–544.

Daugas E, Nochy D, Huong DL, Duhaut P, Beaufils H, Caudwell V, Bariety J, Piette JC, Hill G. Antiphospholipid syndrome nephropathy in systemic lupus erythematosus. *J Am Soc Nephrol.* 2002 Jan;13:42-52.

D'Agati VD, Jennette JC, Silva FG. Atlas of nontumor pathology: Non-neoplastic kidney diseases. Washington: *American registry of pathology-Armed Forces Institute of Pathology*; 2005.

D'Agati VD. Renal disease in systemic lupus erythematosus, mixed connective tissue disease, Sjogren's syndrome, and rheumatoid arthritis. In: Jennett JC, Olson JL, Schwartz MM, Silva FG (eds). Heptinstall's Pathology of the Kidney. Lippincott Williams & Wilkins: Philadelphia, 2007

Ellington KT, Truong L, Olivero JJ. Renal amyloidosis in systemic lupus erythematosus. *Am J Kidney Dis.* 1993 Jun;21:676-8.

Fogo, A. B., & Kashgarian, M. (2012). Diagnostic atlas of renal pathology: A companion to Brenner & Rector's the Kidney, 9th edition. Philadelphia: Elsevier/Saunders.

Gur H, Kopolovic Y, Gross DJ. Chronic predominant interstitial nephritis in a patient with systemic lupus erythematosus: A follow up of three years and review of the literature. *Ann Rheum Dis.* 1987;46:617–23.

Haas M, Kaul S, Eustace JA. HIV-associated immune complex glomerulonephritis with “lupus-like” features: A clinicopathologic study of 14 cases. *Kidney Int.* 2005;67:1381–1390.

Jennette JC. Rapidly progressive crescentic glomerulonephritis. *Kidney Int.* 2003;63:1164-77.

Joshi D, Kumar N, Rai A. Dermatomyositis presenting with rhabdomyolysis and acute renal failure; an uncommon manifestation. *Ann Indian Acad Neurol.* 2009 Jan;12:45-7.

Kashgarian, M., 2002. Lupus Nephritis: Pathology, Pathogenesis, Clinical Correlations and Prognosis. In: Wallace, D.J., Hahn, B.H. (Eds.), *Dubois's Lupus Erythematosus,* sixth ed. Lippincott Williams & Wilkins, pp. 1061-1076.

Kashgarian, M, Hayslett, JP. Renal involvement in systemic lupus erythematosus. in: CC Tisher, BM Brenner (Eds.) *Renal Pathology With Clinical and Functional Correlations.* ed 2. Lippincott, Philadelphia, PA; 1994:442–471.

Kern WF, Silva FG, Laszik ZG, Bane BL, Nadasdy T, Pitha JV. The Nephropathies of Systemic Lupus Erythematosus and Other Rheumatolgic Disorders. In: Kern WF, Silva FG, Laszik ZG, Bane BL, Nadasdy T, Pitha JV, (eds). Atlas of Renal Pathology. 1 st ed. Philadelphia, PA. Saunders, 1999.

Kitridou RC, Akmal M, Turkel SB, et al. Renal involvement in mixed connective tissue disease: A longitudinal clinicopathologic study. *Semin Arthritis Rheum.* 1986;16:135.

Louzada Jr P, Simon MS, Voltarelli JC, Donadi EA: Síndrome do anticorpo antifosfolípide. *Medicina.* 1998;31:305-15.

Meehan SM. Systemic Lupus Erythematosus. In: Colvin RB, ed. *Diagnostic Pathology: Kidney Diseases.* 1st ed. Salt Lake City, Utah: Amirsys, distributed by Lippincott Williams & Wilkins, 2011.

Miyakis S, Lockshin MD, Atsumi T, Branch DW, Brey RL, Cervera R, Derksen RH, DE Groot PG, Koike T, Meroni PL, Reber G, Shoenfeld Y, Tincani A, Vlachoyiannopoulos PG, Krilis SA. International consensus statement on an update of the classification criteria for definite antiphospholipid syndrome (APS). *J Thromb Haemost.* 2006 Feb;4:295-306.

Müller-Höcker J, Schmid H, Weiss M, Dendorfer U, Braun GS. Chloroquine-induced phospholipidosis of the kidney mimicking Fabry's disease: case report and review of the literature. *Hum Pathol.* 2003 Mar;34:285-9.

Nasr SH, D'Agati VD, Park HR, Sterman PL, Goyzueta JD, Dressler RM, Hazlett SM, Pursell RN, Caputo C, Markowitz GS. Necrotizing and crescentic lupus nephritis with antineutrophil cytoplasmic antibody seropositivity. *Clin J Am Soc Nephrol.* 2008 May;3:682-90.

Necrotizing arteritis in a human immunodeficiency virus-infected patient with lupus-like glomerulonephritis. Gyl Eanes Barros Silva, Viviane Alves Leite, Natalino Salgado-Filho, Roberto Cuan Ravinal, José Gabriel Gatti Vergna, Roberto Costa Silva, Márcio Dantas. *Int J Clin Exp Pathol.* 2014;7:464–467.

Nochy D, Daugas E, Droz D, Beaufils H, Grünfeld JP, Piette JC, Bariety J, Hill G. The intrarenal vascular lesions associated with primary antiphospholipid syndrome. *J Am Soc Nephrol.* 1999 Mar;10:507-18.

Petri M, Orbai AM, Alarcón GS, et al.: Derivation and validation of the Systemic Lupus International Collaborating Clinics classification criteria for systemic lupus erythematosus. *Arthritis Rheum.* 2012;64:2677-86.

Singh AK, Ucci A, Madias NE. Predominant tubulointerstitial lupus nephritis. *Am J Kidney Dis.* 1996;27:273-78.

Song D, Wu LH, Wang FM, Yang XW, Zhu D, Chen M, Yu F, Liu G, Zhao MH. The spectrum of renal thrombotic microangiopathy in lupus nephritis. *Arthritis Res Ther.* 2013 Jan 15;15:R12.

Weening JJ, D'Agati VD, Schwartz MM, Seshan SV, Alpers CE, Appel GB, et al. The classification of glomerulonephritis in systemic lupus erythematosus revisited. *Kidney Int*. 2004;65:521-30.

Weening, J.J., D'Agati, I.V., Schwartz, M.M., et al. on behalf of the International Society of Nephrology and Renal Pathology Society Working Group on the Classification of Lupus Nephritis, 2004. The classification of glomerulonephritis in systemic lupus erythematosus revisited. *Kidney Int*. 65, 521-530.

Authors' Contact Information

Dr. Gyl Eanes Barros Silva, MD, PhD
Professor of Department of Pathology
Ribeirão Preto Medical School, University of São Paulo, Brazil
Av. Bandeirantes, 3900, Monte Alegre, Ribeirão Preto-SP, 14049-900
Email: gyleanes@ig.com.br

Roberto Silva Costa, MD, PhD
Professor of Departamento of Pathology
Ribeirao Preto Medical School, University of São Paulo, Brazil
Av Bandeirantes, 3900, Monte Alegre, Ribeirao Preto-SP, 14049-900
Email:rscosta@fmrp.usp.br

Márcio Dantas, MD, PhD
Professor of Division of Nephrology
Ribeirao Preto Medical School, University of São Paulo, Brazil
Av Bandeirantes, 3900, Monte Alegre, Ribeirao Preto-SP, 14049-900
Email:mdantas@fmrp.usp.br

Natalino Salgado Filho, MD, PhD
Professor of Division of Nephrology
Departament of Internal Medicine, Federal University of Maranhão, Brazil
Barão de Itapari, 227 - Centro, São Luís - MA, 65020-070
Email: natalinosalgadofilho@uol.com.br

Stanley de Almeida Araujo, MD
Departamento of Pathology
Federal University of Minas Gerais, Brazil
Av. Alfredo Balena, 190 - sala 5005 - Santa Efigênia,
Belo Horizonte-MG, 30130-100
Email: stanleyaa@gmail.com

Index

A

acid, 25
acute renal failure, 43, 46, 58
acute tubular necrosis, 31, 34
adhesion, ix
adults, 43
advancement, vii
African-American, 21
albumin, 16, 24, 29, 46, 49
amyloidosis, vii, 44, 50, 51, 58
anemia, 45
angiotensin receptor blockers, 12
antibody, 5, 14, 16, 29, 37, 39, 40, 49, 59
anticardiolipin, 39, 40, 41
anticoagulant, 38, 39, 40, 41
antinuclear antibodies, 2
antiphospholipid antibodies, 40, 41
antiphospholipid syndrome, 59
apoptosis, 15
arterial hypertension, 13
artery(s), 1, 35, 37, 39, 40
arterioles, 35, 37, 40, 44
arteritis, 4, 37, 45, 59
arthralgia, 44, 49
arthritis, 5, 58
assessment, 40, 52
asthenia, 46
asymptomatic, 1, 27
atrophy, 16, 17, 29, 30, 35, 38, 40, 46, 47, 48
attachment, ix
authorities, 16
autoantibodies, 23, 43
autoantigens, 32
autoimmune disease(s), 1, 39
autoimmunity, 46

B

basement membrane, ix, x, 14, 27, 33
biopsy, vii, 2, 3, 14, 16, 21, 29, 31, 32, 34, 38, 45, 46, 49, 54
blood, 24, 32, 35, 47
bowel, 50
brain, 39
Brazil, vii

C

cancer, 39
capillary, ix, x, 11, 14, 17, 18, 19, 21, 24, 26, 27, 31, 38
capsule, ix, 27
cardiomyopathy, 53
central nervous system, 5
cerebrovascular disease, 41
children, 2, 43, 45

cholesterol, 12, 49
chronic renal failure, 40
classes, 2, 5, 9, 14, 21, 23, 27, 31, 32, 35, 37
classification, vii, 1, 7, 8, 14, 16, 59, 60
collagen, 31
complement, 36, 51, 52
connective tissue, 43, 57, 58, 59
consensus, 59
contour, x
correlation, vii
corticosteroids, 32, 48
creatinine, 2, 16, 24, 29, 32, 34, 38, 46, 47, 49
crescentic glomerulonephritis, 44, 46, 47, 53, 57, 58
cyclophosphamide, 21
cytokines, 49
cytoplasm, 54, 55

D

deposition, ix, 1, 10, 12, 14, 15, 18, 19, 21, 24, 35, 36, 37, 38, 40, 47, 51
deposits, x, 3, 7, 8, 9, 10, 12, 14, 16, 21, 24, 26, 27, 31, 33, 35, 36, 37, 45, 46, 49, 50, 51, 54
detectable, 10, 23
diabetes, vii, 48
diagnostic criteria, 2, 57
differential diagnosis, 12
diffuse interstitial fibrosis, 46
dilation, 34
direct action, 45
disease progression, 24
diseases, vii, 4, 12, 34, 39, 43, 50, 58
distribution, 12
DNA, 2, 10, 13, 14, 16, 24, 29, 38, 44, 49, 52
drug toxicity, vii, 45
drug-induced lupus, 46, 53
drugs, 12, 34, 35, 47, 49, 53
dyspnea, 44, 47

E

edema, 16, 38, 43, 46, 49
electron, 2, 7, 33, 49
electron microscopy, 2, 7
endocapillary hypercellularity, x, 21
endothelial cells, ix, 14
endothelium, x, 37
enlargement, 38
enzyme, 12
enzyme inhibitors, 12
epithelial cells, 32
epithelium, 15
erythrocytes, 38
etiology, 1
evidence, 27, 39
evolution, 10, 15
excretion, 24, 29

F

Fabry disease, 54, 57
fever, 47, 52
fibrin, ix, 15, 18, 37, 38, 40
fibrosis, ix, 16, 17, 29, 30, 32, 35, 38, 40, 44, 46, 47, 48
fibrous adhesion, ix
fibrous tissue, ix, 15
formation, 15, 18, 32, 57
fragments, 38

G

glomerular nephritis, vii
glomerulonephritis, vii, 1, 3, 8, 12, 14, 21, 23, 26, 29, 43, 46, 47, 53, 57, 58, 59, 60
glomerulus, 1, 8, 19, 43
glucocorticoid, 21
granules, 46
growth, 15
guidance, 54

H

hearing loss, 53
hematocrit, 24
hematuria, 1, 2, 7, 10, 16, 29, 31, 34, 40, 43, 44, 45, 46, 47, 52, 53
hemoglobin, 24
Hispanics, 21
histology, vii, 21
history, vii, 13, 24, 29, 32, 34, 35, 41
host, 53
hue, 15
human, 57, 59
human immunodeficiency virus (HIV), 4, 45, 46, 57, 58, 59
hyaline, 14, 16, 18, 19, 32, 35, 36
hypercellularity, ix, x, 10, 27, 35, 44, 48, 49, 52
hyperplasia, 40, 44
hypertension, vii, 13, 15, 16, 23, 29, 35, 37, 40, 41, 43
hypothesis, 49

I

idiopathic, 23
images, vii
immune function, 51
immune system, 45
immunodeficiency, 57, 59
immunofluorescence, 12
immunoglobulin(s), 12, 51
immunosuppressive agent, 21
immunosuppressive drugs, 12, 35, 49
incidence, 46
individuals, 2
indolent, 23
induction, 21, 34
infarction, 41, 44
infection, vii, 34, 41, 45, 46, 57
inflammation, 16, 30, 31, 33
inflammatory bowel disease, 50
inflammatory disease, 50
injury(s), vii, 2, 3, 4, 10, 15, 27, 35, 45, 49
institutions, vii
interstitial nephritis, 4, 58
intima, 37, 38
ischemia, 38
isoniazid, 53

J

joint pain, 35

K

Karyorrhexias, ix
kidney(s), 1, 15, 30, 31, 39, 46, 47, 58, 59

L

laboratory studies, 29
laboratory tests, 24
learning, viii
lesions, 2, 4, 8, 9, 14, 15, 16, 23, 27, 35, 37, 40, 43, 45, 51, 59
leukocyte(s), ix, 24, 32, 35, 47
leukopenia, 45
light, 11, 12, 24
liver, 39
low-density lipoprotein, 12
lumen, x, 14, 19, 27, 36, 37
lupus, vii, ix, 1, 2, 3, 4, 7, 10, 12, 14, 21, 23, 26, 31, 34, 35, 37, 39, 40, 41, 45, 46, 47, 49, 52, 53, 57, 58, 59, 60
lupus anticoagulant, 37, 39, 40, 41
lupus erythematosus, 57, 58, 59, 60
lupus nephritis, vii, 1, 4, 23, 57, 59
lupus-unrelated renal injury, vii
lymphocytes, 15, 31

M

majority, 10, 14, 29, 35, 41, 51
malignant hypertension, 37
management, 3
matrix, ix, x, 8, 10, 24

media, 44
medication, 12, 41
mellitus, vii, 48
membranoproliferative glomerulonephritis, 12, 21
membranous glomerulonephritis, 23, 26
membranous nephropathy, 43
mesangial cells, ix, x
microscopy, 2, 7, 8
minimal change disease, 44
morbidity, 1
mucoid, 38, 44
myalgia, 44
myelin, 54
myocardial infarction, 41, 44
myocyte, 38
myopathy, 53
myositis, 34, 43

N

National Institutes of Health, 16
necrosis, ix, 3, 4, 15, 16, 18, 21, 31, 34, 37, 38, 44, 46, 47, 48
necrotizing glomerulonephritis, 21
negativity, 10
nephritis, vii, 1, 2, 4, 23, 31, 46, 57, 58, 59
nephrologists, viii
nephropathy, 4, 12, 43, 51, 52, 54, 57, 58
nephrotic syndrome, 1, 2, 10, 13, 43, 45, 49
nervous system, 5
neutrophils, 15, 46
nodules, 35
non-inflammatory necrotizing vasculopathy, vii
nuclei, ix
nucleus, 15

O

occlusion, 17, 27, 38
optical microscopy, 8
organ(s), 1, 45
overlap, 44

P

pain, 34, 35, 39
parenchyma, 30
pathogenesis, 45
pathologist(s), viii, 35
pathology, 58
perinatal, 45
Philadelphia, 58
photosensitivity, 52
plasma cells, 32
plasmapheresis, 46
podocytopathies, vii, 51
polymyositis, 43
prednisone, 21, 27, 54
probability, 14, 16
prognosis, vii, 3, 16, 35, 37
proliferation, ix, 3, 8, 14, 15, 16, 17, 20, 21, 27, 32, 38, 46, 47
proteinase, 46
proteins, 31
proteinuria, 1, 2, 5, 7, 10, 12, 13, 16, 23, 27, 29, 31, 34, 40, 43, 45, 46, 49, 52, 53
proximal tubules, 31
purpura, 21, 37

R

rapidly progressive glomerulonephritis, 1
rash, 5, 52
RBC, 24
receptor, 12
red blood cells, 24, 35, 47
regeneration, 34
renal biopsy, vii, 2, 16, 29, 49
renal dysfunction, 31, 41, 53
renal failure, 14, 16, 37, 40, 43, 45, 46, 58
renin, 12
response, 3, 24, 32, 47, 49
retinopathy, 53
rhabdomyolysis, vii, 4, 34, 57, 58
rheumatoid arthritis, 58
rheumatologists, viii
risk factors, 51

S

scleroderma, 37, 43, 44
sclerosis, 8, 9, 10, 16, 29, 32, 44
sediment, 10, 13, 29
segmental glomerulosclerosis, 4, 45
sepsis, 1
serology, 2, 29
serum, 46, 51
serum albumin, 46
showing, 17, 18, 19, 36, 38
signs, 12, 38, 49
silica, 54
silver, ix, 24
skeletal muscle, 54
skin, 39, 44
steroids, 47
survival, 2, 13, 14, 23, 47
syndrome, 1, 2, 10, 13, 37, 41, 43, 44, 45, 49, 53, 58, 59
synechia, ix
synovitis, 43
systemic lupus erythematosus (SLE), vii, 1, 2, 4, 10, 23, 24, 29, 31, 32, 34, 40, 41, 43, 44, 45, 46, 47, 48, 49, 50, 51, 53, 54, 57, 58, 59, 60
Systemic Lupus International Collaborating Clinics (SLICC), 2, 59

T

therapy, 12, 21, 27, 46, 48, 54
thrombocytopenic purpura, 37
thrombosis, 39
thrombotic microangiopathy, vii, 43, 45, 59
thrombus, ix, 38, 39
tissue, ix, 15, 43, 57, 58, 59
toxicity, vii, 45, 54
transformation, 2, 5
transverse section, 40
treatment, 2, 5, 12, 16, 27, 47, 49, 50, 53, 54

U

uniform, 24
United States, 16
urinalysis, 16, 32, 44
urine, 13, 16, 35, 44

V

validation, 59
vascular occlusion, 41
vascular wall, 37, 40
vasculitis, vii, 4, 37
vasculopathy, vii, 4, 36, 37
vein, 39
vessels, 36, 44
viral infection, 41
virus infection, 57

W

Washington, 58
white blood cells, 24
withdrawal, 53
World Health Organization (WHO), 1, 4, 7, 8, 9